STRONG & STILL: MENTAL FITNESS FOR MEN OVER 40

Normalizing Emotional Self-Care for Men with Grit.

NICCI BROCHARD
&
DR. BEN CHUBA

STRONG & STILL: MENTAL FITNESS FOR MEN OVER 40

Normalizing Emotional Self-Care for Men with Grit.

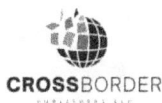

CROSSBORDER

New York, London, Quebec

Also published by Nicci Brochard and Dr. Ben Chuba

1. How To Be Alone Without Feeling Lonely: *An Easy Guide To Enjoying Company With Yourself, Growing Strong Mentally, And Surviving Rejection.*

2. The Power Of Your Subconscious Mind And Emotions: *Techniques To Resist Negativity, Stay Focused And Positive, And Find Happiness In Daily Activities.*

3. From paycheck to payday: *How To Make Money Last Longer In Your Pocket, Understand The Mind, Measure Money, And Build Everlasting Wealth.*

4. When Decluttering Is Not An Option: *Techniques To Reimagine & Reinvent Your Space And Yourself With Less Stress, Anxiety, And Freedom From Perfectionism.*

5. Conversations Between Women: *A Comprehensive Guide To Decipher The Female Code, Think Like A Woman, And Build A Lasting Relationship With Her.*

6. Conversations Between Men: *A Comprehensive Guide To Decipher The Male Code, Think Like A Man, And Build A Lasting Relationship With Him.*

7. Social Savviness For Teens And Young Adults: *A Modern Guide To Overcoming Social Media Traps, Anxiety, Peer Pressure, And The Fear Of Missing Out.*

CONTENTS

INTRODUCTION

The Myth of the Unbreakable Man

For generations, the societal narrative surrounding masculinity has glorified the idea of the "unbreakable man." This myth suggests that men, particularly as they age, must maintain an image of stoic strength, invulnerability, and relentless perseverance. Emotions, vulnerability, and mental well-being were seen as weaknesses to be hidden or suppressed, especially as men entered their 40s and beyond. This outdated notion has perpetuated harmful stereotypes and prevented countless men from seeking the help they need to maintain not just their physical health but also their emotional and mental fitness.

However, this myth is not only unrealistic—it's harmful. It paints an impossible picture of manhood, one that forces men to silently bear the weight of their struggles, suffering in isolation and keeping their emotions locked away. As men enter their 40s, they often face significant transitions—whether in their careers, family dynamics, health, or personal goals. These years are full of challenges, but they are also the beginning of depth, not the end. Rather than fearing these changes, men can embrace this stage of life as an opportunity to refine their mental resilience, build a deeper sense of self-awareness, and develop a new form of strength that includes emotional agility and mental wellness.

In this book, *Strong & Still: Mental Fitness for Men Over 40*, we aim to normalize emotional self-care for men, especially those over 40, and redefine what it means to be strong. This journey is about discovering a new model of mental fitness that doesn't ask men to deny their emotions or suppress their vulnerability, but instead invites them to cultivate stillness alongside their grit. Strength no longer means the absence of vulnerability; it means the ability to adapt, reflect, and grow, even when faced with life's inevitable challenges.

Breaking the Stigma Around Men's Mental Health

The stigma surrounding men's mental health has been a longstanding issue, preventing many men from seeking help or expressing their emotions. Mental health, especially in the context of emotional vulnerability, was traditionally seen as something reserved for women, or as something weak that "real men" should not have to deal with. In the past, men's emotional struggles were often dismissed or minimized, with phrases like "man up" or "push through it" being commonly used to discourage emotional expression.

As a result, many men internalize the idea that seeking help for mental health issues is a sign of failure or weakness. This can lead to denial, isolation, and an inability to process feelings of anxiety, depression, or stress. However, in reality, ignoring emotional health only increases mental strain, chronic stress, and can even lead to physical ailments such as heart disease, high blood pressure, and sleep disorders.

It is essential to break this cycle and start conversations that normalize mental health care for men. Mental health struggles are not signs of weakness; they are simply part of the human experience. By breaking the stigma, men can begin to openly engage in self-care, seek professional support when needed, and learn new strategies to cope with the pressures of life. Therapy, mindfulness, emotional expression, and self-compassion can be incredibly beneficial to men's mental fitness, just as much as exercise is to physical fitness.

Why 40+ Is Not the Beginning of the End—It's the Beginning of Depth

Turning 40 often comes with societal messages about aging, midlife crises, and the inevitable decline of energy, health, and ambition. These messages are not only untrue but deeply limiting. In reality, the age of 40 and beyond is an opportunity to embrace a more authentic version of masculinity—one that integrates emotional depth, wisdom, and mental resilience.

For men, turning 40 is often the point at which they begin to reflect on their lives—the choices they've made, the relationships they've formed, and the legacy they wish to create. It is a time for reinvention and recalibration. It's not about slowing down or retreating into complacency; it's about gaining clarity and recognizing that the best is yet to come. At this age, men have lived through enough experiences to understand what really matters and can begin to make choices that align with their values and purpose.

Rather than seeing aging as a limitation, men over 40 can embrace it as a time to deepen their understanding of themselves and their emotional needs. This is a phase where emotional growth and maturity become key assets, allowing men to let go of superficial expectations and focus on what truly nourishes their mind, body, and spirit. Mental fitness at this stage is about learning to manage the emotional and psychological complexities of life, and finding ways to stay balanced while continuing to pursue goals and live with vitality.

The Balance of Strength and Stillness: A New Mental Fitness Model

True strength is not the absence of vulnerability; it is the ability to remain grounded, focused, and adaptable in the face of adversity. A **new model of mental fitness** for men over 40 combines both **strength and stillness**, recognizing that emotional resilience doesn't come from pushing harder or ignoring pain, but from creating a **balanced approach** to life that integrates **action** and **reflection**.

The idea of balancing strength with stillness is not about doing less; it's about doing things with purpose and intention. It's about learning to pause, to reflect, and to be aware of one's emotional and mental state. A mentally fit man does not rush to fix everything or power through every challenge without considering the emotional toll it may take. Instead, he creates space for self-care, emotional expression, and mental recovery—he understands that true strength includes the capacity to take a step back, regroup, and recalibrate when needed.

The balance of strength and stillness can be seen as a form of mental resilience—a strength that allows men to navigate challenges with a calm and grounded approach. It involves integrating self-compassion into their mental fitness practices, letting go of perfectionism, and embracing their emotional landscape with acceptance and openness. This model encourages men to be whole, recognizing that mental fitness is not only about performance, but about building emotional tools that help them thrive in every area of life.

CHAPTER 1

MIDLIFE CHECK-IN – WHERE ARE YOU, REALLY?

Introduction

Hitting the age of 40 can be a defining moment for many men—a threshold between youth and maturity, between chasing ambitions and contemplating legacy. It's often seen as a marker for midlife, a period where physical, mental, and emotional changes start to occur. But for many men, it's also when they find themselves facing an **invisible wall**, an emotional and existential crossroads that demands attention and introspection. The midlife check-in is a necessary moment for reflection, assessment, and realignment—an opportunity to evaluate not just where you are in life but where you want to be in the years ahead.

At 40, many men experience what some might call a midlife crisis—a period of intense introspection, self-doubt, or dissatisfaction. They start to question the meaning and direction of their lives, often driven by internal and external pressures. Yet, this time doesn't have to be one of panic or regret. Instead, it can be an opportunity for growth, clarity, and transformation. In this chapter, we'll explore how to assess your emotional and psychological well-being, recognize signs of stress and dissatisfaction, and most importantly, engage in reflection without shame. It's about mapping your internal terrain and understanding the roots of your emotions and actions.

Assessing Your Emotional Dashboard: Stress, Satisfaction, and Regrets

The first step in the midlife check-in is understanding your **emotional dashboard**—that internal gauge that tells you how you're really feeling. Too often, men put on a mask, adhering to the expectations of being stoic and strong, which makes it harder to recognize the signals of emotional unrest. As you move through life, **stress**, **satisfaction**, and **regrets** accumulate like traffic on a road that's barely holding together. By pausing and checking in on these key areas, you can begin to see whether you're moving in the right direction or if there are roadblocks that need to be cleared.

Stress: The Silent Drain

Stress is one of the most powerful and invisible forces that affect men in midlife. In the earlier years of adulthood, stress may have been easy to ignore, powered by ambition, excitement, or sheer determination. But around 40, stress often begins to feel more profound. The accumulation of responsibilities, unresolved emotional baggage, and personal expectations can start to take their toll.

- The Weight of Responsibility: For many men, the pressure of providing for their families, advancing in their careers, and managing personal relationships becomes more overwhelming by the age of 40. At this point, the challenges are no longer just about getting ahead—they're about maintaining balance. Financial pressures, the need to support children, aging parents, or a significant other can contribute to chronic stress. This is compounded by the fear of financial insecurity or job stagnation that some men experience as they enter their 40s.

- **Physical Symptoms of Stress:** Chronic stress often manifests in physical symptoms. Men in their 40s may notice an increase in tension headaches, back pain, digestive issues, sleep disturbances, or an increased susceptibility to illness. Stress can also take an emotional toll, leading to feelings of anxiety, irritability, or depression.

Real-life Example:

- John, a 45-year-old father of two, found himself increasingly irritable at work and at home. He had been the sole provider for his family for many years, working long hours and juggling multiple responsibilities. His stress was so high that it started affecting his sleep, and he found himself easily frustrated over minor issues. It wasn't until he took time off to reflect that he recognized how much of his stress was tied to a lack of work-life balance and the pressure of meeting high expectations.

Satisfaction: What's Filling Your Cup?

Satisfaction is another key metric on your emotional dashboard. By midlife, men often find themselves questioning the level of fulfillment they're experiencing in various aspects of their lives: career, relationships, health, personal growth, and social connections. Satisfaction isn't just about achievement—it's about feeling a sense of purpose and connection to what you do.

- Career Satisfaction: At 40, many men have invested significant time and effort into their careers. Yet, some may find themselves stuck in a career that no longer aligns with their passions, interests, or values. They may feel unfulfilled, underappreciated, or burned out. The drive for success can overshadow deeper personal fulfillment, leading to dissatisfaction and a desire for change.

- Relationship Satisfaction: Another area of life that often comes under scrutiny during midlife is relationships—whether it's a marriage, friendships, or family connections. Men at this stage may experience disconnect or frustration with the people closest to them. If relationships have been neglected or taken for granted, they may be strained, leading to dissatisfaction and emotional tension.

Real-life Example:

- Tom, a 42-year-old executive, was making more money than ever and had reached a senior position at his company. Yet, he felt empty inside. Despite his career success, he felt no passion for his job anymore, and his personal relationships had deteriorated because of the long hours and lack of attention to his emotional needs. After taking a personal retreat, Tom realized that he had prioritized external achievements over internal happiness. This realization led him to shift his focus to activities and relationships that provided a deeper sense of fulfillment.

Regrets: The Weight of Unsaid Words and Unlived Dreams

Regrets are the silent burden of the midlife experience. Men over 40 often reflect on what they haven't done, what they missed, or the opportunities they didn't seize. The weight of these regrets can be overwhelming if they are left unaddressed. The critical question is: are your regrets about past mistakes, or are they about missed opportunities that you still have the power to change?

- Missed Opportunities: At midlife, it's common to feel regret over opportunities that weren't pursued—whether it was starting a business, traveling the world, or making bold personal decisions. The regret can become a nagging feeling, pulling you away from the present moment and creating emotional distress.

- Regret of Relationships Lost: Another area of regret involves relationships. Men may regret losing touch with friends, neglecting family members, or failing to invest in their marriage. These regrets often carry deep emotional weight and can lead to feelings of guilt or loneliness.

- Internal Regrets: These are regrets that come from a place of self-criticism or self-doubt—not living up to your potential, not taking risks, or staying in a comfort zone that prevented growth. These types of regrets can lead to self-shaming and a sense of hopelessness if not addressed.

Real-life Example:

- David, a 49-year-old lawyer, began reflecting on his life after a health scare. He regretted not pursuing his dream of writing, which he had abandoned in his 20s for the stability of a legal career. The fear of failure had kept him from acting on his creative passion. However, instead of succumbing to regret, David decided to start writing again, channeling his feelings into a blog. By doing so, he began to reconcile with his past and embrace the joy of living authentically, no matter his age.

Why Many Men Hit an "Invisible Wall" Around 40

The concept of hitting an "invisible wall" around the age of 40 is common among men. This midlife transition isn't a sudden event; it's a gradual accumulation of thoughts, feelings, and changes in physical and emotional states. The invisible wall represents a crisis of identity—a time when men feel compelled to question who they are, where they've been, and where they are going. It's a time when external pressures meet internal reflections, and the inevitable process of aging brings a deeper awareness of mortality and the passage of time.

Several factors contribute to this "invisible wall" effect:

- Physical Changes: Around 40, the body begins to undergo significant changes—energy levels fluctuate, metabolism slows down, and recovery from physical activity becomes slower. These changes often bring about the realization that youth and invincibility are fading, which can lead to feelings of loss or discomfort.

- Shift in Values and Priorities: At midlife, many men begin to reevaluate their life's purpose and priorities. What once seemed important—career success, financial achievement—may no longer feel as satisfying or meaningful. The drive for achievement may give way to a longing for balance, happiness, and connection.

- Cultural Expectations: Society places heavy expectations on men, especially in their 40s. Men are often expected to be financially successful, emotionally stable, and constantly achieving. When men fail to meet these expectations, or when they feel overwhelmed by the pressure to do so, they may feel trapped behind an invisible wall.

Real-life Example:

- Michael, a 44-year-old IT manager, hit his "invisible wall" after facing a significant health crisis. His demanding job, long hours, and neglect of his health led to a heart attack. This event forced him to confront the reality of aging and the fragility of life. He started re-evaluating his life choices, realizing he had neglected his emotional health and relationships in pursuit of career success. By slowing down and reconnecting with his values, Michael was able to break through the wall and begin a healthier, more fulfilling life.

Reflection Without Shame: Mapping Your Internal Terrain

A critical part of this midlife check-in is learning how to reflect without shame. Reflection can often be a painful process, as it brings up both pride and regret. However, the goal is not to dwell on mistakes or perceived failures but to map your internal terrain—to understand where you are emotionally, psychologically, and spiritually.

- Self-Awareness: Self-reflection requires the courage to look inward without judgment. It means acknowledging the areas where you've grown and the areas where you need to improve. It's about understanding your emotional landscape, identifying the sources of your stress and satisfaction, and creating a vision for the future that aligns with your true self.

- No Shame, Just Growth: Reflection should not be a shameful process. It's about learning from past experiences and applying those lessons moving forward. Shame can block growth, while self-compassion opens the door to new possibilities.

Real-life Example:

- Steve, a 47-year-old project manager, began to journal as a way to reflect on his experiences. He had long struggled with perfectionism and self-doubt, but journaling helped him unpack those feelings. Over time, Steve found that the process of reflection without shame allowed him to forgive himself for past mistakes and begin making changes that led to greater personal fulfillment and inner peace.

Conclusion

The midlife check-in is an essential part of the emotional growth process for men over 40. By taking the time to assess your emotional dashboard, recognizing the stress, satisfaction, and regrets that shape your life, you can move forward with clarity and purpose. The "invisible wall" many men face is not a permanent barrier but an opportunity to pause, reflect, and recalibrate. Reflection without shame is key to navigating this period with intention, self-compassion, and growth.

Through this introspective process, men can reclaim their mental health and emotional well-being, stepping into the second half of life

CHAPTER 2

THE PRESSURE COOKER – SILENT STRESS IN MIDLIFE

Introduction

Midlife can be a time of great transition, with many men experiencing what feels like a pressure cooker of responsibilities. Around the age of 40, the responsibilities of life seem to accumulate, and with it, a silent stress that is often overlooked. The external pressures of a demanding career, the internal demands of raising children, the evolving dynamics of marriage, and the added weight of caring for aging parents can create a storm of emotional and mental strain. This silent stress doesn't always show up in obvious ways; it's often a low, constant hum that simmers beneath the surface, leaving men to feel overwhelmed but unable to pinpoint the source.

The unspoken weight of midlife can have a profound impact on mental health. In many cases, the stressors are compounded, creating a pressure cooker effect. The expectation that men must continue to perform at high levels, both personally and professionally, while juggling these competing demands, can lead to burnout, quiet depression, and emotional fatigue. These are not always the obvious, outward signs of stress, but they are just as damaging, affecting not only the man's well-being but his relationships, work, and overall quality of life.

In this chapter, we'll explore the pressures that come with midlife, how they manifest silently, and the impact they have on a man's emotional and mental health. We'll discuss the concept of silent stress, the difference between pressure and purpose, and how to recognize the signs of burnout, quiet depression, and emotional fatigue. Understanding these challenges is the first step toward reclaiming balance, mental clarity, and emotional well-being in midlife.

1. Unspoken Weight: Career, Kids, Marriage, Aging Parents

As men approach their 40s, the unspoken weight of balancing multiple responsibilities begins to take a toll. Each area of life—career, family, relationships, and caregiving—carries its own set of pressures. These responsibilities can often feel like a series of unrelenting expectations placed on one's shoulders, with little opportunity for release.

Career Pressures: The Drive for Success and Stability

At this stage, many men find themselves in the midst of their career peak—a time when they've gained significant experience, yet are still striving for professional recognition, financial stability, or career progression. There's a constant drive to perform at the highest level, to meet deadlines, solve problems, and maintain job security. However, the constant grind of trying to keep up with workplace expectations, especially as the work environment becomes more demanding and competitive, can lead to significant stress.

- Unrealistic Expectations: As men grow older, their roles often become more complex, and the expectations from both employers and employees increase. There's the expectation to mentor younger colleagues, to perform at a high level, and to continue innovating. These pressures can leave little room for self-care, creativity, or relaxation.

- Fear of Stagnation: In the corporate world, midlife can be a time of reckoning for many men. There may be a growing fear of being passed over for promotions or being replaced by younger talent. These feelings of insecurity can lead to stress and a sense of professional dissatisfaction, even when outwardly everything seems to be progressing.

Real-life Example:

- Eric, a 45-year-old lawyer, had worked hard to build his practice and achieve financial stability. However, as he neared his mid-40s, he began to feel the weight of increasing expectations—more clients, more pressure to bill hours, and the fear of stagnation in a competitive industry. Despite his achievements, he often found himself lying awake at night, wondering if he was really fulfilling his true potential or simply going through the motions for the sake of security.

Raising Children: The Emotional and Financial Demands

As men approach midlife, they often find themselves in the midst of parenthood, with children at varying stages of development. Raising children, particularly teenagers or young adults, brings unique emotional and financial demands.

- Emotional Investment: Being present for children's emotional, academic, and social growth requires significant time and attention. Many men find themselves acting as emotional providers, trying to guide their children through the challenges of growing up while balancing their own emotional needs.

- Financial Strain: The cost of raising children—especially during the high school and college years—can be a major source of stress. Many fathers feel the pressure to provide for their children's education, extracurricular activities, and future goals. This financial strain can lead to feelings of guilt and responsibility that weigh heavily on a man's shoulders.

Real-life Example:

- Dave, a 42-year-old father of two teenagers, found himself balancing the pressures of work with the financial demands of supporting his children's education and extracurricular activities. His kids were excelling academically, but Dave was overwhelmed by the idea of managing their college tuition while keeping up with mortgage payments. The emotional toll was significant, leaving him feeling physically and mentally exhausted.

Marriage and Relationships: Maintaining Connection Amidst the Chaos

The demands of marriage and intimate relationships can also feel like an added weight during midlife. As men reach their 40s, they may find themselves struggling to maintain intimacy, emotional connection, and communication with their spouse or partner.

- Evolving Roles: Marriage dynamics often change as men approach midlife. Partners may be dealing with different stages of life—whether it's the challenges of raising children, dealing with aging parents, or adjusting to empty-nest syndrome. These changes can create tension and emotional disconnect if not addressed.

- Emotional Distance: With the pressures of work and family life, men may find themselves emotionally distant from their partner. The constant juggling act can lead to neglecting the emotional needs of the relationship, leading to feelings of isolation or resentment.

Real-life Example:

- Tom, a 46-year-old business executive, and his wife, Julie, had been together for over 20 years. However, Tom's career demands and focus on providing for the family began to take a toll on their marriage. Julie began to feel emotionally disconnected, while Tom, exhausted from work and family pressures, withdrew even further. They eventually sought couples counseling, realizing that they both needed to invest more in their emotional connection, despite the busyness of life.

Caring for Aging Parents: The Burden of Caregiving

In midlife, many men face the added responsibility of caring for aging parents, which can bring emotional, physical, and financial burdens. As parents age, they often experience health declines, requiring care and support. Men in their 40s are often caught between caring for their own children and supporting their aging parents.

- Emotional Toll: The emotional weight of seeing a parent age, become ill, or lose independence can be overwhelming. Men may feel guilty for not being able to do more, or they may struggle with the idea of losing their parents.
- Practical Strain: The practicalities of caregiving—arranging doctor's appointments, managing medication, and ensuring that parents are comfortable—can drain emotional and physical energy.

Real-life Example:

- Mark, a 48-year-old man, found himself managing his father's health crisis while still caring for his teenage children. His father's declining health meant frequent doctor visits, handling medical bills, and providing emotional support. Mark found himself becoming more anxious and stressed, as he struggled to balance these responsibilities with his work and family life. His emotional fatigue became apparent in his interactions with others, and he eventually sought therapy to help manage the pressure.

2. Understanding Burnout, Quiet Depression, and Emotional Fatigue

The overwhelming pressure that comes from juggling multiple responsibilities often leads to burnout, quiet depression, and emotional fatigue. These conditions are particularly dangerous because they can be subtle and difficult to recognize until they have already taken a toll on a man's mental and physical health.

Burnout: The Silent Saboteur

Burnout is the state of being emotionally, mentally, and physically exhausted due to prolonged stress. Men in midlife, particularly those with demanding careers, families to support, and aging parents to care for, are at significant risk for burnout.

- Signs of Burnout: Symptoms of burnout can include chronic fatigue, irritability, lack of motivation, depersonalization, and a feeling of disconnection from work or relationships. Men who experience burnout often feel as though they are running on empty, unable to recharge despite taking time off.

- Impact on Relationships: Burnout often affects men's relationships, as they become emotionally unavailable, withdrawn, or impatient. The frustration and exhaustion from work and other pressures spill over into personal interactions.

Real-life Example:

- Brian, a 45-year-old teacher, was on the verge of burnout after years of working long hours, managing school responsibilities, and caring for his family. Despite taking vacations, he couldn't shake the feeling of emotional emptiness. His personal relationships began to suffer, and he struggled to find meaning in his work. Brian eventually sought support from a therapist, who helped him identify signs of burnout and develop coping strategies, such as setting better boundaries and prioritizing self-care.

Quiet Depression: The Hidden Struggle

Depression in midlife often manifests quietly, without the overt signs seen in younger years. Men may experience a lack of enthusiasm, disconnection from joy, and feelings of hopelessness. Unlike younger individuals, men in midlife may not exhibit typical signs of depression like tearfulness or overt sadness. Instead, they may internalize these feelings, leading to chronic stress and emotional isolation.

- Internalizing Emotions: Men are often conditioned to suppress their emotions, making it difficult to recognize when depression is taking hold. Quiet depression often presents as chronic dissatisfaction, irritability, or a feeling of emptiness, but it may not always be accompanied by sadness.

- Impact on Health: Left unchecked, quiet depression can affect both physical and mental health. It can lead to sleep disturbances, weight changes, and reduced energy levels, further exacerbating the emotional burden.

Real-life Example:

- John, a 50-year-old sales manager, had been feeling increasingly detached from his work and personal life. He wasn't experiencing the sadness typically associated with depression but felt a deep sense of emptiness. After a series of sleepless nights and declining energy, he recognized that he was experiencing quiet depression. Seeking help from a counselor allowed John to open up about his emotions and begin addressing the underlying causes of his dissatisfaction.

Emotional Fatigue: The Unseen Drain

Emotional fatigue is the result of prolonged stress and emotional strain. Men in midlife, especially those facing multiple competing responsibilities, often experience exhaustion not just from physical activity but from the constant emotional demands they face.

- Symptoms of Emotional Fatigue: Men experiencing emotional fatigue may feel disconnected, withdrawn, or apathetic. They may feel overwhelmed by even small tasks, struggle to connect with others, and feel numb to life's joys.
- Coping Mechanisms: Often, men will turn to unhealthy coping mechanisms, such as excessive work, alcohol, or disengagement. These mechanisms offer short-term relief but worsen emotional fatigue in the long run.

Real-life Example:

- Nick, a 47-year-old father and project manager, noticed that he had been feeling emotionally drained for months. Despite getting adequate sleep, he could not shake the sense of exhaustion. His relationships felt distant, and his performance at work was slipping. Nick realized that the emotional weight of caring for his children, managing a stressful job, and taking on household responsibilities had left him emotionally fatigued. He began working with a coach to develop healthier emotional boundaries and ways to restore his energy.

3. The Difference Between Pressure and Purpose

Midlife is a time of reflection, and it's critical to differentiate between pressure and purpose. Pressure is often externally driven—the weight of others' expectations, societal standards, and responsibilities. Purpose, on the other hand, is internally driven—it's about living in alignment with one's values and finding meaning in what you do.

- Pressure: Pressure is a constant force that drives you to perform, meet deadlines, and achieve. It comes from external sources and can lead to stress, burnout, and emotional fatigue.

- Purpose: Purpose is the driving force that aligns your work and personal life with your values and goals. When you have a clear sense of purpose, even the most demanding challenges feel meaningful.

The key to navigating midlife stress is learning to shift from external pressure to internal purpose. When you are aligned with your true values, you can face challenges with clarity, motivation, and resilience.

Real-life Example:

- James, a 44-year-old executive, felt suffocated by the constant pressures of his job. However, after reflecting on his life and work, he realized that he had been chasing external validation—the need for success and approval. He decided to reconnect with his true passions, pursuing projects that aligned with his values and brought a sense of purpose to his life. This shift not only relieved his stress but also reignited his passion for his career and relationships.

Conclusion

In midlife, men face a unique set of challenges that can lead to silent stress, burnout, and emotional fatigue. By understanding the unspoken weight of responsibilities and differentiating between pressure and purpose, men can begin to navigate the complexities of this phase with greater clarity and emotional resilience. Recognizing the signs of burnout, quiet depression, and emotional fatigue is the first step toward regaining control and finding balance. Midlife does not have to be a crisis; it can be a time of reflection, growth, and reinvigoration.

CHAPTER 3

EMOTIONAL FITNESS – WHAT IT IS, WHY IT MATTERS

Introduction

In a world that increasingly demands more from us, the importance of emotional fitness has never been clearer, especially for men navigating the complexities of midlife. Historically, emotional well-being has often been sidelined in favor of physical fitness or professional success, with men particularly being conditioned to prioritize "toughness" over "tenderness." However, emotional fitness, much like physical fitness, is essential for overall health, well-being, and success in life. The ability to manage stress, process emotions, and bounce back from setbacks is not merely a "nice-to-have" trait but a critical life skill, especially for men over 40, who may face personal, professional, and familial challenges at unprecedented rates.

This chapter seeks to redefine emotional fitness in practical terms. Instead of relying on therapeutic jargon or abstract concepts, we will break down what emotional fitness means for men, why it is crucial, and how to integrate emotional strength into everyday life. Just as one would go to the gym to build physical muscles, emotional strength requires intentional effort, consistency, and practice. It is through this lens that we can explore the concepts of grit, resilience, recovery, and reflection—the cornerstones of emotional fitness that empower men to live their lives with balance, clarity, and adaptability.

1. Defining Mental/Emotional Fitness for Men (Not Therapy-Speak)

When we talk about emotional fitness, we're discussing the ability to understand, regulate, and apply emotions in ways that promote healthy relationships, personal growth, and overall well-being. This is not a concept limited to mental health professionals or therapy rooms. Instead, it is a practical skill set that anyone—especially men—can develop and use in their day-to-day lives.

Emotional fitness can be described as a man's capacity to:

- Identify and understand his emotions: Acknowledging what you're feeling is the first step toward emotional fitness. This is about recognizing your emotional state in real-time and understanding what triggers specific responses. For example, feeling frustration at work or resentment in a relationship should be acknowledged without judgment, so it can be addressed in a healthy way.

- Regulate emotions effectively: Emotional fitness involves the ability to manage emotions instead of being controlled by them. This doesn't mean suppressing feelings or pretending they don't exist. Rather, it's about having the tools and strategies to manage emotional reactions in high-stress situations. It means knowing how to calm yourself down when angry, seek clarity when confused, and find joy when life feels mundane.

- Apply emotional intelligence in interactions: Emotional fitness also means understanding how emotions affect relationships, communication, and decision-making. Men with emotional fitness can navigate conflicts with others more easily, build stronger bonds, and create positive outcomes in both personal and professional settings.

Real-life Example:

- Steve, a 42-year-old architect, was known for his intense work ethic and dedication to his career. However, this commitment often led to emotional outbursts, particularly with his colleagues and family members. One day, during a team meeting, Steve realized he was reacting to stress in a way that alienated his coworkers. Instead of denying his emotions, Steve acknowledged his frustration and sought to understand why he felt that way. By learning emotional regulation techniques like deep breathing and taking brief breaks to recalibrate, Steve was able to navigate workplace stress more calmly and improve his relationships at work.

This practical emotional fitness is not about cultivating an overly Zen persona or repressing feelings; it's about developing the emotional awareness and resilience needed to handle life's challenges while staying grounded.

2. The Grit-Based Model: Resilience, Recovery, and Reflection

Emotional fitness for men is not only about feeling good but also about being strong enough to withstand life's inevitable blows. Much like physical fitness, emotional fitness involves grit— a combination of resilience, recovery, and reflection. These core components provide the framework for developing the emotional strength necessary to thrive in the face of adversity.

Resilience: Bouncing Back Stronger

Resilience is the ability to bounce back after experiencing stress, failure, or disappointment. It's about adapting to change and maintaining your focus even when the world around you feels chaotic. In midlife, men may encounter challenges such as job changes, health issues, or evolving family dynamics. Resilience allows men to face these challenges head-on, without losing their sense of self or purpose.

Resilience isn't just about enduring hardship; it's about learning from it. Resilient men view adversity as an opportunity to develop strength and wisdom, not as a reason to give up or give in. This mindset shift is what allows individuals to thrive during difficult times.

- Building Mental Toughness: To develop resilience, men need to work on strengthening their mental toughness. This involves accepting setbacks as a natural part of life and learning how to overcome them with a positive mindset. Mental toughness also means having the emotional fortitude to keep moving forward despite setbacks.

Real-life Example:

- Gary, a 46-year-old business owner, faced a significant loss when his business was forced to close after the economic downturn. Instead of sinking into despair, Gary chose to view the closure as an opportunity to pivot. He used his experience as a foundation to start a new business that better aligned with his passions and values. His resilience not only led to personal growth but also to a thriving new venture.

- Recovery: The Importance of Rest and Renewal

- While resilience is about bouncing back, recovery is about giving yourself the space and time needed to rest and renew after stress or hardship. Recovery is a key part of emotional fitness, yet it is often overlooked in the pursuit of achievement or success. In midlife, men often feel the pressure to perform without pause, but recovery is essential for emotional well-being.

- Recovery doesn't just mean resting physically; it's about engaging in activities that restore emotional and mental balance. It could involve practices like:

- Self-care routines: Regular practices that nurture the body and mind, such as exercise, meditation, and healthy eating.

- Hobbies and creative outlets: Engaging in activities that bring joy and fulfillment without any external pressure or goals.

- Quality sleep: The foundation of emotional and physical recovery is sleep. It's during sleep that the brain processes emotions, regenerates energy, and recharges the body for the next day.

Men often underestimate the power of recovery, thinking that rest is for the weak. In reality, recovery is the key to sustained **emotional fitness**. It's about giving yourself permission to **pause** and **recharge**, so you can face future challenges with strength and clarity.

Real-life Example:

- Michael, a 49-year-old financial advisor, was known for his relentless work ethic. However, he found himself increasingly burnt out and disconnected from his family. After discussing his exhaustion with a friend, he realized that he needed to prioritize recovery. Michael began taking weekends off, scheduling regular breaks during the day, and investing time in mindfulness practices. Over time, this recovery routine helped him regain his focus, energy, and sense of purpose.

Reflection: Learning from Experience

Reflection is the process of looking back on past experiences to gain insight and wisdom. Emotional fitness requires that men engage in regular reflection to understand their emotions, behaviors, and growth. Without reflection, it's difficult to learn from mistakes or recognize patterns in your emotional responses.

Reflection can take many forms, from journaling to mindful introspection. The key is to be honest with yourself and approach your emotions with curiosity, not judgment. Reflection helps men:

- Identify patterns in emotional responses, such as stress triggers or unhealthy coping mechanisms.
- Understand their needs and make adjustments to live a more balanced, intentional life.
- Set future goals based on insights gained from past experiences.

Real-life Example:

- Paul, a 43-year-old high school teacher, began journaling to process the emotional stress he felt at work. Through his reflections, he realized that much of his stress came from his desire to please others—his students, their parents, and his colleagues. He started to reflect on what really mattered in his life and how he could set boundaries without feeling guilty. His ability to reflect allowed him to set healthier boundaries and make positive changes in his life.

3. Just Like the Gym—Emotional Strength Needs Reps

Just like physical fitness, emotional fitness requires consistent effort. You wouldn't expect to build physical strength by lifting weights once or twice a year, and the same goes for emotional strength. To be emotionally fit, men need to practice self-awareness, emotional regulation, and resilience regularly. This is where the concept of emotional reps comes in—just as you would go to the gym to build physical strength, you need to engage in consistent emotional fitness exercises to develop mental and emotional resilience.

- Daily Practices: Emotional fitness requires regular exercises, such as mindfulness meditation, stress management, and emotion regulation techniques. These daily practices help build emotional resilience over time.

- Growth Mindset: As with physical fitness, emotional growth comes from challenging yourself and embracing discomfort. Engaging in difficult conversations, confronting emotional triggers, and taking on new emotional challenges will help strengthen your emotional muscles.

- Consistency: Emotional fitness doesn't work unless you commit to regular practice. The more consistent the effort, the stronger your emotional muscles become, allowing you to navigate life's challenges with confidence and calmness.

Real-life Example:

- Daniel, a 44-year-old sales manager, noticed that he struggled to keep his emotions in check during stressful meetings. Instead of letting frustration or anger take over, he began practicing deep breathing exercises and journaling each morning to set a calm tone for the day. Over time, these emotional reps helped him stay composed during tense situations and improved his relationships with colleagues.

Conclusion

Emotional fitness is an essential component of living a balanced and fulfilling life, especially for men over 40. By developing resilience, prioritizing recovery, and engaging in regular reflection, men can strengthen their emotional well-being and learn to navigate life's challenges with clarity and strength. Just like physical fitness, emotional strength requires **consistent practice**. By investing time in building emotional muscles, men can face stress and adversity with confidence, creating a life of purpose, **emotional clarity**, and inner peace. Through this process, they can redefine what it means to be emotionally strong—not by suppressing their emotions but by learning to manage them with skill and resilience.

REWRITING THE MAN CODE – DROP THE TOUGH GUY ACT

Introduction

For generations, men have been conditioned to uphold a strict "man code"—an unspoken set of rules dictating how men should behave, think, and express themselves. This code often includes emotional armor like stoicism, silence, and emotional suppression. While these traits were once seen as necessary for survival and success, particularly in the face of challenges or adversity, the reality is that they often do more harm than good. In the modern world, especially as men reach midlife, there is a growing recognition that these outdated ideas of masculinity are not only limiting but also emotionally and mentally destructive.

The idea of being the "tough guy"—a man who suppresses his emotions, avoids vulnerability, and never shows weakness—may have once been a marker of strength. However, it is becoming increasingly clear that this model of masculinity is flawed, particularly as men age and encounter the complexities of midlife. The truth is, real strength doesn't come from bottling up emotions or pretending to be invulnerable; it comes from embracing vulnerability, expressing emotions in healthy ways, and learning to redefine masculinity for today's world.

In this chapter, we will unpack the emotional armor that many men have spent years constructing—armor built from stoicism, silence, and emotional suppression. We will explore the damaging effects of these behaviors and the importance of rewriting the man code for modern midlife. The journey involves redefining what it means to be masculine, recognizing that true strength is rooted not in avoidance of feelings, but in the ability to be open, authentic, and vulnerable. Through this process, men can embrace a more holistic and healthy version of masculinity—one that promotes emotional well-being, genuine connection, and mental fitness.

1. Unpacking Emotional Armor: Stoicism, Silence, Suppression

The traditional "man code" encourages men to put on a metaphorical suit of armor in order to withstand the emotional storms that life inevitably throws their way. This armor consists of three primary components: stoicism, silence, and emotional suppression. While these traits may have served men well in certain situations, they have also contributed to emotional isolation, poor mental health, and strained relationships.

Stoicism: The Myth of Emotional Detachment

Stoicism—the ancient philosophy that emphasizes endurance of pain or hardship without the display of feelings—has often been used as a model for masculine behavior. For many men, stoicism became a way of life. The idea was to mask pain and emotion in the pursuit of strength and self-control. The prevailing belief was that men should endure suffering without letting it affect them emotionally or psychologically.

- The Problem with Emotional Detachment: While stoicism can offer resilience in difficult times, it comes with significant drawbacks. Suppressing emotions leads to emotional bottling—a phenomenon where unresolved feelings, such as grief, anger, and fear, accumulate over time, only to erupt later in unhealthy ways. This emotional suppression not only harms mental health but also damages relationships. Men who adhere too rigidly to stoic principles may find themselves emotionally distant from their spouses, children, or friends, unable to connect on a deeper, more vulnerable level.

- Real-life Example: John, a 47-year-old lawyer, had always prided himself on being stoic. He never let his emotions get the best of him at work or home. However, after a series of professional setbacks, John found himself increasingly irritable, isolated, and unfulfilled. The emotional armor he had built to protect himself began to take a toll on his relationships and his overall happiness. Eventually, John sought therapy, realizing that his attempts at stoicism had led to emotional burnout and a sense of disconnection from those around him.

Silence: The Pressure to Be Silent in the Face of Struggles

Silence is another key element of the emotional armor that many men adopt. The idea that "real men don't talk about their feelings" or "man up" when facing emotional difficulties is deeply ingrained in our cultural narrative. Men are often taught that speaking openly about personal struggles is a weakness, and that silence is the appropriate response in times of emotional distress.

- The Cost of Silence: The silence that many men adopt in response to emotional struggles can create a sense of emotional isolation. Men may feel as though they are carrying their burdens alone, unable to reach out for support or even acknowledge the difficulties they face. This silence can lead to a lack of emotional intimacy in relationships and an inability to connect with others on a deeper level. Additionally, emotional silence often exacerbates mental health issues such as anxiety, depression, and stress.

- Real-life Example: Tom, a 45-year-old business executive, kept his emotional struggles bottled up for years. He rarely spoke to his wife or friends about his fears, insecurities, or the stress from his demanding job. Over time, his silence created a rift in his relationship with his wife, who felt disconnected from him. Tom's reluctance to open up ultimately led to anxiety and emotional numbness, which affected his work performance and mental health. Only after attending a support group for men did Tom realize that speaking about his challenges allowed him to release pent-up emotions and rebuild his relationships.

Emotional Suppression: Denying Feelings for the Sake of Strength

Many men believe that to be strong, they must suppress their emotions altogether. The idea of "toughing it out" and denying the presence of negative emotions is a core component of the traditional "man code." Emotions such as sadness, fear, or vulnerability are often perceived as weaknesses that must be hidden.

- The Dangers of Suppressing Emotions: Emotional suppression may seem effective in the short term, but it has long-term consequences. Suppressed emotions often find their way to the surface in unhealthy ways—through anger, outbursts, exhaustion, or chronic stress. Suppressing emotions also deprives men of the opportunity to process and heal from their experiences. Over time, this can lead to emotional disconnection, strained relationships, and even physical ailments such as headaches, stomach problems, and high blood pressure.

- Real-life Example: Alex, a 50-year-old engineer, spent most of his adult life suppressing emotions. He avoided confronting his feelings of sadness following his father's death and fear about his career stagnation. Instead of expressing his emotions, he threw himself into work, pushing through the pain. Eventually, his health began to deteriorate—he developed insomnia and digestive issues. Through therapy, Alex learned that acknowledging and expressing his emotions was the key to healing and restoring his overall health.

2. Redefining Masculinity for Modern Midlife

As men reach midlife, the concept of masculinity often comes under scrutiny. In the face of aging, shifting societal norms, and changing priorities, many men find themselves questioning what it means to be a "real man" at this stage of life. The traditional notion of masculinity—marked by emotional suppression, stoicism, and silence—no longer resonates with many men as they seek deeper emotional fulfillment and connection.

Breaking Down the Old Model of Masculinity

The traditional model of masculinity tells men that they must be stoic, emotionally reserved, and self-sufficient. This model often values physical strength over emotional intelligence, independence over collaboration, and action over reflection. While these qualities may have served men well in certain situations, they are inadequate for the complex emotional and psychological landscape that many men encounter in midlife.

In midlife, men are often faced with questions about their purpose, legacy, and emotional fulfillment. The old model of masculinity, based on toughness and self-reliance, can feel out of place in a world that demands emotional literacy, healthy relationships, and the ability to embrace vulnerability. Modern masculinity is not about abandoning strength; rather, it's about redefining what strength means.

Embracing a New Definition of Strength

Modern masculinity calls for a redefinition of strength—one that incorporates vulnerability, empathy, and emotional openness. True strength is not about hiding emotions or avoiding vulnerability; it's about having the courage to show up as you are, acknowledging your fears and struggles, and expressing your needs in healthy ways. This is the strength that leads to genuine connections, personal growth, and emotional well-being.

- Strength in Vulnerability: Vulnerability is often seen as a weakness, but in reality, it is one of the most powerful forms of strength. Vulnerability means being open to emotional experiences, being honest with yourself, and allowing yourself to be seen without fear of judgment. Vulnerability is not about being weak; it's about having the courage to face your emotions head-on and showing others that it's okay to do the same.

- Emotional Intelligence as a Strength: Modern men are increasingly recognizing that emotional intelligence—the ability to understand, regulate, and express emotions—is a key component of true strength. Men who develop emotional intelligence are better equipped to navigate relationships, handle stress, and lead with empathy and understanding.

Real-life Example:

- Chris, a 44-year-old teacher, started to reevaluate his understanding of masculinity after experiencing a period of emotional burnout. He had always prided himself on being strong and self-sufficient, but he realized that his refusal to open up about his feelings had taken a toll on his relationships. By embracing vulnerability, Chris learned to express his emotions more freely, improving his relationships with his colleagues and family and finding greater personal fulfillment.

3. Strength in Vulnerability: What That Really Means

The concept of strength in vulnerability may seem counterintuitive at first. Many men have been taught to view vulnerability as a weakness—something that undermines their masculinity. However, embracing vulnerability is actually a hallmark of true emotional strength.

Vulnerability as Emotional Courage

Vulnerability involves showing emotional openness and honesty—traits that require great courage. It's not about being emotionally exposed or fragile; it's about authentically expressing yourself, even when it feels uncomfortable. Vulnerability allows men to connect with others on a deeper level, creating more meaningful relationships. It also enables men to acknowledge their feelings of fear, grief, insecurity, or hurt, and to process these emotions in a healthy way.

- The Courage to Be Seen: Vulnerability is the courage to be seen as you are, flaws and all. It's about letting go of the need for perfection and embracing your authentic self. Vulnerability invites deeper connection, as it shows others that it's okay to be imperfect and to face challenges openly.

Real-life Example:

- Richard, a 50-year-old father, struggled with vulnerability for most of his life. He had always been the "strong, silent" type. However, after a health scare, Richard realized that his emotional withdrawal had distanced him from his children and spouse. He began to open up more, sharing his fears and insecurities with his family. Over time, this vulnerability allowed him to build stronger, more honest relationships and feel more connected to those he loved.

Conclusion

Rewriting the "man code" means letting go of the outdated ideals of stoicism, silence, and emotional suppression that have long been associated with masculinity. True strength comes not from hiding emotions, but from embracing vulnerability, expressing feelings, and living authentically. By reimagining what it means to be a man in midlife, men can foster deeper emotional connections, achieve greater mental resilience, and create a more fulfilling life. In this chapter, we've explored how dropping the tough guy act can lead to true emotional fitness, enabling men to live with purpose, connection, and strength—all while embracing the full range of their emotional experiences.

CHAPTER 5

STRESS, ANXIETY & THE MIDLIFE MIND

Introduction: Understanding the Emotional Landscape of Midlife

As men approach and move through their 40s, the midlife transition can trigger a complex web of emotions and experiences, including stress and anxiety. While these emotions are a natural part of the human experience, they manifest in distinct ways during midlife and require a new approach for management and understanding. For many men, stress and anxiety are no longer fleeting concerns; they become persistent, underlying forces that affect both mental health and overall well-being. In this chapter, we'll explore how stress shows up differently in men after 40, why anxiety is not a sign of weakness but rather an important signal, and how men can learn to recognize, name, and manage these emotions with skill and resilience.

In midlife, the traditional notion of "being tough" or "pushing through" can exacerbate emotional distress. Men who have spent much of their lives suppressing feelings of stress and anxiety may find themselves overwhelmed in ways they didn't anticipate. This chapter will focus on the unique experience of stress and anxiety in midlife, the importance of embracing vulnerability, and the development of mental fitness tools to confront and manage these emotions effectively.

By the end of this chapter, you will gain clarity on why stress and anxiety in midlife are normal, how they show up in your daily life, and practical strategies you can use to navigate and manage these emotional experiences with maturity and insight.

1. How Stress Shows Up Differently After 40

Stress manifests in different ways throughout a person's life, and the way it impacts men in their 40s differs from how it might affect younger individuals. The combination of life responsibilities, physical changes, and societal pressures creates a unique emotional landscape for men in midlife.

Physical Stress: A New Kind of Wear and Tear

In your 40s, the body begins to experience physical changes that can compound feelings of stress. These changes are often not drastic but are subtle yet cumulative. You may notice a slower metabolism, changes in energy levels, and less efficient recovery from physical activity. These physical signs of aging can create underlying stress that compounds emotional and mental strain.

- Decreased Physical Resilience: As men age, their bodies don't bounce back as quickly from exertion, illness, or even emotional challenges. This means that stress from work, relationships, or financial pressures can also manifest physically—whether through fatigue, headaches, muscle tension, or trouble sleeping. The body, which was once a reliable source of strength, begins to demand more attention and self-care. This can create stress on its own, as men struggle to maintain the same level of performance they had in younger years.

- Sleep Disruptions: As men reach their 40s, sleep can become a significant stressor. Hormonal changes, changes in work/life balance, and mental preoccupation with aging or future goals can lead to difficulties in getting restful sleep. Chronic sleep deprivation exacerbates stress, heightens anxiety, and decreases the body's ability to recover physically and mentally. Poor sleep can also trigger a vicious cycle, increasing the likelihood of stress and emotional burnout during the day.

Real-life Example:

- Brian, a 47-year-old IT consultant, noticed that after he turned 40, his energy levels dropped significantly. He was working long hours at his job, which required constant mental focus and problem-solving. After work, he would often have trouble winding down and sleeping. The lack of rest, combined with the constant mental strain, began to manifest as muscle tension, headaches, and mood swings. Over time, Brian realized that he needed to pay attention to his physical health—eating better, exercising regularly, and improving his sleep hygiene to mitigate stress.

Emotional Stress: Increased Personal and Professional Pressures

Midlife is often characterized by an intersection of personal and professional responsibilities, leading to heightened stress. Men over 40 often face pressures that are not present in earlier years, including career stagnation, parenting teenagers, and the caregiving of aging parents. These added responsibilities can feel like an emotional overload, causing stress to accumulate and, in some cases, become unmanageable.

- Career Pressures: Many men experience pressure to be successful in their careers, especially in midlife. At 40, men may feel the weight of having to continue proving themselves in their professional lives, particularly if they are experiencing job changes, facing workplace ageism, or transitioning into different roles. There's often a desire to remain relevant, secure financial stability, and maintain leadership positions, which can feel overwhelming.

- **Family Pressures:** Men in their 40s often carry the responsibility of being a provider, but also a caretaker. As children become teenagers or young adults, the financial and emotional support they require may increase. At the same time, many men in this stage also begin caring for aging parents. Balancing the needs of both their children and their parents can create significant emotional stress. The weight of responsibility can be compounded by the feeling of losing control over their own time and energy.

Real-life Example:

- David, a 49-year-old engineer, was dealing with the stress of a career transition after his company underwent a restructuring. At the same time, he had to help his teenage daughter navigate her high school challenges while also assisting his elderly father with daily tasks. David often found himself feeling spread too thin, unable to devote enough time or energy to any one responsibility. The emotional toll of juggling these roles led him to experience increased stress and anxiety, often manifesting as irritability and a sense of helplessness.

Mental Stress: The Midlife Identity Crisis

In midlife, mental stress is not just about external pressures— it also arises from internal questions about identity, purpose, and legacy. Men often start to reflect on the decisions they've made, the goals they've yet to accomplish, and the meaning of their achievements. Midlife is often a time of personal reevaluation, which can create a mental crisis.

- Self-Doubt and Imposter Syndrome: As men approach midlife, they may begin to experience self-doubt and feelings of inadequacy. This is especially true if their career or personal life has not progressed in the way they envisioned. The pressure to be successful at midlife, coupled with the sense of time running out, can create a significant amount of mental stress. Men may feel like they're not living up to their potential or that they are falling behind.

- Fear of Aging: Aging, while natural, brings with it a fear of obsolescence. Men may begin to worry about their health, physical appearance, or mental sharpness. These concerns are not only about vanity but also about a deep-seated fear of losing relevance or becoming invisible in society.

Real-life Example:

- Chris, a 45-year-old creative director, was beginning to question his career choices after 20 years in the industry. Despite outward success, he started to feel unfulfilled and doubted whether he had made the right career choices. He also began to notice physical changes and worried about his health. This led to mental stress, as Chris found himself questioning his life's direction, feeling stagnant in both his career and personal life.

2. Anxiety Isn't Weakness – It's a Signal

Anxiety often gets a bad rap, particularly in men's health discussions. It's easy to dismiss anxiety as a sign of weakness or inadequacy, but this is far from the truth. Anxiety is a natural response to stress, uncertainty, and the pressures of life, and it is not inherently bad or a sign that something is wrong. In fact, anxiety is a signal—a message from your mind and body that something needs attention.

The Role of Anxiety: A Natural Alarm System

Anxiety serves as an internal alarm system, alerting us to potential threats or challenges. However, in today's fast-paced, high-pressure world, anxiety can become a constant companion, often triggered by work stress, family obligations, or personal expectations. While acute anxiety can be beneficial (helping us focus or react to threats), chronic anxiety can become overwhelming, especially when the source of anxiety is unclear or constantly changing.

- Recognizing Anxiety as a Signal: The first step in managing anxiety is recognizing it as a signal rather than a weakness. When anxiety arises, it's important to assess what it's telling you. Are you feeling overwhelmed by your workload? Do you need to set better boundaries? Is your body trying to tell you to slow down? Recognizing anxiety as a natural response rather than a failure allows men to take proactive steps to manage their emotional health.

- Common Anxiety Triggers in Midlife: In midlife, anxiety often stems from concerns about aging, career progression, and personal identity. Financial stability, health fears, and family dynamics are significant sources of anxiety for many men in their 40s.

Real-life Example:

- Mark, a 48-year-old teacher, often felt anxious in social situations. However, he realized that his anxiety was linked to his desire for approval from others. This realization allowed him to understand that his anxiety was not a sign of personal weakness, but a response to his internal fear of judgment. By identifying the source of his anxiety, Mark was able to address his need for external validation and reduce his anxiety by focusing on his own values.

3. Tools to Recognize, Name, and Manage Stress and Anxiety Like a Pro

Managing stress and anxiety in midlife requires a combination of awareness, self-compassion, and practical strategies. Emotional fitness doesn't mean eliminating stress or anxiety; it's about developing the **tools** and **skills** to manage these emotions in a healthy and proactive way.

Tool 1: Mindfulness and Awareness

Mindfulness is the practice of being present in the moment, fully aware of your thoughts, feelings, and sensations without judgment. By cultivating mindfulness, men can become more attuned to their emotional state, noticing when stress or anxiety begins to build up.

Mindful Breathing: Simple breathing techniques, such as deep diaphragmatic breathing, can help reduce the physiological symptoms of anxiety. Focusing on the breath can ground you in the present moment and reduce mental chatter.

Real-life Example: Tim, a 44-year-old software developer, found that taking five-minute mindfulness breaks during work helped him manage stress. By practicing deep breathing and focusing on the present moment, he was able to refocus his energy and reduce feelings of overwhelm.

Tool 2: Cognitive Reframing

Cognitive reframing involves changing the way you think about a stressful situation. It means shifting from negative thinking to a more balanced, solution-focused perspective.

- Positive Self-Talk: Instead of internalizing anxiety and self-doubt, practice positive affirmations and self-compassionate statements. Remind yourself that it's okay to feel anxious or stressed—it's a natural part of life, and you have the ability to handle it.

Tool 3: Regular Physical Activity

Exercise is one of the best ways to manage stress and anxiety. Physical activity helps release endorphins, which naturally improve mood and reduce tension.

- Exercise as Stress Relief: Whether it's a daily walk, lifting weights, or participating in a favorite sport, regular exercise is an essential tool in managing stress and anxiety.

Real-life Example:

- Rick, a 46-year-old carpenter, discovered that running each morning helped him manage his stress levels. Not only did it provide an outlet for his physical energy, but it also gave him a sense of clarity and calm, reducing his overall anxiety.

Conclusion

Midlife can be a period of emotional reckoning, but it is also a time of great opportunity for personal growth and mental clarity. Stress and anxiety are natural components of the human experience, and they show up differently as men enter their 40s. The key to navigating this stage of life is recognizing stress and anxiety as signals rather than weaknesses. By embracing mindfulness, cognitive reframing, and regular physical activity, men can develop the emotional fitness needed to manage stress and anxiety like a pro. Emotional health is not a destination—it's a practice that requires attention, intention, and consistency.

CHAPTER 6

RELATIONSHIPS, RAGE & RESENTMENT

Introduction

Midlife is a period of profound change, and it often brings with it a deep reassessment of relationships. Whether it's with a spouse, children, friends, or colleagues, men in their 40s experience a unique mix of emotional turbulence and relationship challenges. Issues like irritability, withdrawal, and emotional distance often surface, creating tension and disconnect. While many men may attribute these feelings to the pressures of work or personal challenges, they are also rooted in deeper emotional processes that are often ignored or suppressed.

As men enter midlife, they often find themselves confronting unresolved emotional issues and unaddressed personal frustrations, leading to feelings of rage and resentment. These emotions, if left unchecked, can erode the fabric of key relationships, making it difficult to experience true intimacy and emotional connection with loved ones.

However, this period of emotional upheaval also presents an opportunity for growth and change. Through self-awareness, communication, and conflict resolution, men can work to heal the rifts in their relationships, let go of grudges, and approach emotional conflicts with clarity. In this chapter, we will explore how midlife irritability, withdrawal, and emotional distance manifest, the often-overlooked emotional labor of marriage, fatherhood, and friendship, and, most importantly, how to move beyond resentment and manage conflict in a way that fosters growth, understanding, and connection.

1. Midlife Irritability, Withdrawal, and Emotional Distance

For many men, irritability becomes a significant feature of midlife. As men approach 40 and beyond, the pressures of work, family, health, and aging can combine to create a sense of frustration that often manifests as irritability. This irritability might be directed inward, leading to feelings of frustration with oneself, or outward, affecting those closest to them.

Irritability: The Overlooked Symptom of Emotional Strain

Irritability in midlife is often rooted in emotional stress, and it typically surfaces when men are unable to fully express or manage their emotions. When personal or professional stress mounts and there's no healthy outlet for release, irritability becomes a common response.

- Signs of Midlife Irritability: Men in midlife may find themselves snapping at family members or colleagues, becoming easily frustrated by minor annoyances, or retreating into themselves when faced with challenges. This behavior is often a form of emotional suppression—a signal that the person is struggling to process underlying feelings like stress, inadequacy, or fear.

- Why Men Experience More Irritability in Midlife: The changes associated with aging, such as shifts in career, financial concerns, health challenges, and changes in family dynamics, can all contribute to a heightened sense of irritability. As a result, many men feel a sense of loss or uncertainty that manifests through frustration.

Real-life Example:

- David, a 47-year-old father of two, noticed that he had become increasingly irritable with his family. Small things, like a forgotten chore or a disagreement about a family event, would trigger an explosive reaction. David's irritability stemmed from his work stress, where he was under constant pressure to meet deadlines. He had not realized that his frustration at work was bleeding into his home life, creating emotional distance between him and his wife. After seeking therapy, David realized that his irritability was a symptom of unresolved emotional strain, and learning to express his feelings constructively helped him reconnect with his family.

Withdrawal: Emotional Disconnection as a Defense Mechanism

In addition to irritability, many men in midlife begin to withdraw emotionally from relationships. This withdrawal can take various forms: physical withdrawal from family events, mental disengagement from conversations, or an overall sense of emotional distancing.

- Emotional Disengagement: For some men, emotional withdrawal becomes a way to protect themselves from feeling vulnerable or overwhelmed. They may distance themselves from loved ones to avoid confrontation, criticism, or difficult conversations.
- The Cost of Withdrawal: While withdrawal may feel like a way to cope, it ultimately creates emotional disconnect and loneliness. In relationships, particularly in marriages and

close friendships, withdrawal leads to a lack of communication, understanding, and intimacy. Over time, this emotional distance can erode the quality of relationships, causing hurt feelings and misunderstandings.

Real-life Example:

- John, a 50-year-old manager, found himself withdrawing from his wife after several years of marriage. The demands of his career and concerns about his health had led him to retreat into his own world, spending long hours at work or in front of the TV to escape emotional intimacy. His wife, feeling neglected, became frustrated and distant as well. It wasn't until John acknowledged his emotional withdrawal and opened up about his feelings that they were able to start repairing their relationship. This process required vulnerability and honest communication, two aspects of emotional fitness that John had been avoiding.

2. The Hidden Emotional Work of Marriage, Fatherhood, and Friendship

In midlife, men often find themselves shouldering a tremendous amount of emotional labor in their relationships, though it may not always be visible or acknowledged. This is the emotional work involved in maintaining a marriage, raising children, and nurturing friendships—work that is often invisible but essential for the health and stability of these relationships.

Marriage: The Emotional Labor of Keeping the Connection Alive

Marriage is one of the most important relationships in a man's life, yet it also requires ongoing emotional effort. At midlife, many men are faced with challenges that test the strength of their relationship: empty nest syndrome, midlife crises, financial stress, or health issues. The emotional work required to maintain a healthy marriage during this time is often underestimated.

- Emotional Maintenance: In midlife, emotional labor in marriage is about more than just communication; it's about emotional maintenance—keeping the connection alive and ensuring both partners feel heard, understood, and supported. Men often feel the weight of this work, especially if they are the primary emotional provider in the relationship. When a man neglects this emotional labor, it can lead to resentment and disconnection.

Real-life Example:

- Tom, a 48-year-old man in a long-term marriage, began to notice his relationship with his wife was becoming strained. He had been so focused on his career that he had neglected the emotional maintenance of their marriage. His wife, feeling emotionally disconnected, began to withdraw, and they found themselves arguing more frequently. By acknowledging the hidden emotional labor involved in marriage, Tom took proactive steps to reconnect with his wife, including scheduling regular date nights and being more emotionally available.

Fatherhood: The Emotional Demands of Parenting

As men enter midlife, they may have children who are transitioning into adolescence or adulthood. Fatherhood during this time brings emotional challenges that differ from earlier years. The emotional work of parenting shifts from providing basic care to navigating the complexities of raising independent, emotionally intelligent children.

- The Struggles of Parenting Teenagers: Fatherhood during midlife often involves managing the tensions of raising teenagers—dealing with emotional outbursts, helping children navigate relationships and education, and balancing their growing independence with the desire to remain involved in their lives.

- The Burden of Expectations: Men may also feel the emotional pressure to support their children financially and emotionally, especially as they begin to approach adulthood. Fathers are often expected to be a source of strength, yet they may feel ill-equipped to address their children's complex emotional needs.

Real-life Example:

- Chris, a 45-year-old father, struggled with his relationship with his teenage son. His son was rebelling and pushing boundaries, which left Chris feeling frustrated and helpless. Chris began to recognize that his emotional withdrawal and avoidance of conflict were only making things worse. He sought advice from a counselor and learned how to engage with his son in a compassionate and patient way, leading to a stronger, more open relationship.

Friendship: Navigating the Emotional Needs of Male Friendships

Friendships among men often evolve in midlife. As men juggle career, family, and personal health, maintaining deep, meaningful friendships can feel challenging. Many men find that they don't have the time or energy to nurture these relationships, leading to a sense of emotional isolation.

- The Emotional Disconnect in Male Friendships: Men are often socialized to view friendships as more transactional than emotional. They are encouraged to compete rather than connect emotionally, making it difficult for them to bond with friends in meaningful ways. However, the emotional labor of maintaining friendships is necessary for personal well-being. Friendships offer support, validation, and a sense of belonging—emotional needs that men must actively cultivate.

Real-life Example:

- James, a 49-year-old lawyer, realized that over the years, he had lost touch with his close friends. The demands of work and family left little time for socializing. After some self-reflection, James recognized that his isolation was contributing to feelings of stress and loneliness. He reached out to a few close friends and made an effort to spend more time with them, allowing for emotional connections and mutual support to flourish.

3. Letting Go of Grudges and Managing Conflict with Clarity

At midlife, men often carry emotional baggage from past relationships or experiences. Grudges, resentment, and unresolved conflicts can have a profound impact on their emotional well-being and relationships. The inability to release these negative emotions can create emotional distance and perpetuate cycles of frustration and anger. However, letting go of grudges is a key component of emotional fitness.

The Power of Forgiveness

Letting go of resentment and learning to forgive—both others and oneself—is essential for emotional health. Forgiveness doesn't mean condoning harmful behavior; it means releasing the emotional hold that past hurts have over your present life.

- Releasing Emotional Baggage: Grudges often hold us in a state of emotional stagnation, preventing us from moving forward. By letting go of anger and resentment, men can create the emotional space necessary for growth, healing, and connection.

Real-life Example:

- Mark, a 47-year-old marketing executive, had been holding onto resentment toward his former boss, who had passed him over for a promotion years ago. This grudge weighed heavily on him, affecting his mental clarity and self-esteem. After years of harboring resentment, Mark realized that he needed to forgive and move on. He acknowledged that the grudge was not serving him and chose to focus on his present and future, letting go of the past.

Conflict Resolution: Managing Disagreements with Clarity

Conflicts in midlife—whether in marriage, friendships, or professional life—are often magnified by the emotional baggage that accompanies them. Men often approach conflict with a desire to win, avoid, or suppress, rather than addressing the issue with clarity and calmness.

- Healthy Conflict Resolution: In midlife, men can benefit from embracing healthy conflict resolution strategies— such as active listening, emotional regulation, and empathetic communication. These tools allow men to address issues without escalating the emotional tension, fostering greater understanding and connection.

Real-life Example:

- Scott, a 50-year-old doctor, often found himself arguing with his wife over trivial issues. Through counseling, Scott learned how to manage conflicts in a healthier way. He began listening actively to his wife's concerns, expressing his feelings without blame, and approaching disagreements with a problem-solving mindset. This shift in approach led to a significant improvement in his marriage and emotional health.

Conclusion

Midlife can bring a heightened sense of emotional and relational stress, especially when it comes to dealing with irritability, withdrawal, and the emotional demands of marriage, fatherhood, and friendship. By recognizing and addressing these challenges, men can navigate this stage of life with greater emotional intelligence and clarity. Letting go of grudges, embracing vulnerability, and learning to manage conflict with empathy and understanding are key steps in building stronger, more fulfilling relationships. In doing so, men can improve their emotional health, repair damaged connections, and cultivate the resilience necessary for navigating midlife with purpose and strength.

CHAPTER 7

THE SILENT STRUGGLE – DEPRESSION IN MEN

Introduction

Depression is often thought of as an emotional state characterized by sadness, hopelessness, and despair. While these symptoms are certainly present for many people experiencing depression, the manifestation of depression in men often looks different. For many men, depression doesn't appear as sadness. Instead, it shows up as numbness, escape behaviors, burnout, and even rage. This distinction is crucial because it means that men, especially those in midlife, may not even recognize that they are suffering from depression. Worse still, society's reluctance to acknowledge male vulnerability can prevent men from seeking the help they need.

This chapter aims to explore how depression manifests in men, particularly those over 40, and offer insight into why it's often so hard to recognize. We will delve into the behaviors and emotional states that often accompany male depression—such as numbness, escape behaviors, low-grade rage, and burnout—and how they contribute to the silent struggle that many men face. We'll also discuss the importance of self-awareness and the steps toward healing, from recognizing the signs to seeking professional help.

By understanding depression in men in its full context, this chapter aims to provide men with the tools and language to recognize their emotional pain, begin their healing journey, and ultimately reclaim their mental fitness.

1. What Male Depression Actually Looks Like (Hint: Not Always Sadness)

The most common misconception about depression is that it's primarily about feeling sad. While sadness is an important component of depression for some, the symptoms that many men experience are often far more subtle, making it harder for them to identify their struggles. For men, depression often manifests in indirect ways that are more acceptable or easier to ignore— especially in a culture that often discourages men from expressing vulnerability.

Emotional Numbness

For many men, depression feels like **numbness**. Instead of overwhelming sadness, men may feel emotionally **disconnected**, unable to experience joy, fulfillment, or even sorrow. This emotional flatness can be just as debilitating as sadness itself.

- Loss of Interest: Men in midlife often experience a loss of interest in things they once enjoyed—whether that's hobbies, work, or socializing. What once brought excitement or satisfaction no longer feels engaging, and the man may struggle to muster up any emotional response to daily life.

- Disconnection: Numbness can also result in emotional disconnection from loved ones. Men may find themselves unable to connect with their spouse, children, or friends, leading to a sense of isolation and loneliness. This disconnection can further exacerbate depression, making the person feel even more distanced from the world around them.

Real-life Example:

- David, a 46-year-old father and software engineer, found himself withdrawing from his wife and children despite having a stable family life. He noticed that he didn't feel happy during family outings anymore and even struggled to get excited about personal projects he once loved. After months of feeling emotionally numb, David realized that he wasn't just experiencing burnout—he was likely suffering from depression. His inability to feel anything, whether it was joy or sadness, was a key symptom of his condition.

Escape Behaviors

In many cases, men experiencing depression resort to escape behaviors as a way to cope with their emotional pain. These behaviors often involve avoidance or distraction, as the individual attempts to flee from the overwhelming emotional state they are experiencing.

- Substance Abuse: Men may turn to alcohol, drugs, or other substances as a way to numb their feelings or escape reality. While these substances may provide temporary relief, they exacerbate the underlying emotional issues, leading to a cycle of dependency and deeper depression.
- Excessive Work or Hobbies: Some men dive into work, exercise, or hobbies to distract themselves from their emotional struggles. They may overwork, throw themselves into a new project, or immerse themselves in physical pursuits as a way to avoid confronting their emotions.

- Technology and Media: Another escape behavior is turning to screen time—whether binge-watching TV shows, playing video games, or scrolling through social media. These distractions offer temporary relief but do little to address the root causes of the emotional turmoil.

Real-life Example:

- Mark, a 49-year-old businessman, began drinking more heavily after his company went through a downsizing. He used alcohol as a way to cope with the stress and disappointment from the layoffs, but it led to further emotional withdrawal. His friends noticed he was isolating himself, and his family grew concerned about his increasing reliance on alcohol. Mark eventually realized that his drinking was a coping mechanism for deeper feelings of hopelessness and loss that he had not yet acknowledged.

Burnout: The Chronic Strain of Midlife

While burnout is not exclusive to men, it is particularly prevalent in midlife, when men are balancing multiple roles and responsibilities. Burnout in men often presents as a deep sense of emotional and physical exhaustion. It is the result of prolonged stress—often in the workplace or in family life—that hasn't been properly managed.

- Physical Symptoms: Men experiencing burnout may feel constantly drained, experience insomnia, or have headaches and muscle tension. These physical symptoms often overlap with the signs of depression and are often ignored or dismissed as part of normal stress.

- Emotional Exhaustion: Emotionally, burnout can leave a man feeling detached from his work or relationships. He may lose his sense of purpose or fulfillment, viewing his responsibilities as burdens rather than meaningful endeavors.

Real-life Example:

- Michael, a 45-year-old doctor, had been working in an intense hospital environment for over 15 years. He had always prided himself on his ability to handle stress, but after years of long shifts, constant decision-making, and a lack of personal time, Michael began feeling completely drained. He no longer felt the passion for his work that he once had. Instead of addressing the underlying cause, he pushed through the exhaustion, thinking it was just a phase. His performance declined, and his relationships began to suffer. Only after acknowledging his burnout did Michael begin to take steps to prioritize self-care and set healthier boundaries at work.

Low-Grade Rage: The Hidden Emotion of Male Depression

Anger, particularly low-grade rage, is another common manifestation of depression in men. Unlike the outward sadness that is often associated with depression, men often internalize their emotional struggles, which can turn into chronic irritation, frustration, or rage.

- The Connection to Depression: This anger is often the result of unaddressed emotional pain—feelings of powerlessness, helplessness, or injustice. Since many men have been conditioned not to express vulnerability, this pain is often channeled into anger, making it difficult for them to understand or articulate their feelings.

- Impact on Relationships: When unchecked, this anger can manifest in arguments with loved ones, outbursts at work, or passive-aggressive behavior. This can create tension and conflict in relationships, which only deepens the sense of isolation and frustration.

Real-life Example:

- Alan, a 50-year-old teacher, found himself increasingly frustrated with his students and colleagues. He snapped during meetings and was short with his family at home. Alan initially thought he was simply under stress, but his constant irritation pointed to deeper emotional turmoil. Through counseling, he learned that his anger was actually a cover for deeper feelings of inadequacy and fear about his future. Addressing the root causes of his anger helped Alan reconnect with his family and regain a sense of balance in his work life.

2. Steps Toward Light: From Self-Awareness to Professional Help

Recognizing depression is the first step toward healing. Self-awareness is essential, as it allows men to acknowledge their emotional struggles and take proactive steps to address them. Men often avoid seeking help because of societal expectations or pride, but understanding that emotional fitness requires external support is vital for long-term recovery.

Self-Awareness: The Foundation of Healing

The first step in managing depression is recognizing and acknowledging it. This requires self-awareness—an ability to honestly assess one's emotional state without judgment. It's about noticing when irritability, withdrawal, or low-grade rage begin to interfere with daily life.

- Self-Reflection: Journaling, mindfulness, and introspection are tools that can help men explore their emotions and identify the root causes of their depression. By regularly checking in with themselves, men can become more attuned to their emotional states, making it easier to recognize when things are getting out of hand.

- Talk to Trusted Individuals: Sharing feelings with trusted friends, family, or mentors can be a powerful tool for building self-awareness and finding support. Sometimes, simply talking about feelings of frustration or sadness can help break the isolation that often accompanies depression.

Seeking Professional Help: Acknowledging the Need for Support

If depression is severe or persistent, seeking professional help is a critical step. Therapy, medication, and support groups can provide tools and resources that promote healing. Therapy offers men a safe space to express their feelings, identify patterns, and develop coping strategies.

- Therapy Options: Cognitive-behavioral therapy (CBT), psychotherapy, and other therapeutic models can help men address the underlying causes of depression and develop healthier ways to cope with emotions.

- Medication: In some cases, medication may be prescribed to help regulate mood and reduce the symptoms of depression. While medication is not a cure, it can provide the necessary support for men to begin working through their emotional challenges.

Real-life Example:

- Eric, a 45-year-old accountant, had been living with low-grade depression for several years. He had always dismissed his symptoms as "normal stress," but after his relationships with his colleagues and family began to suffer, he decided to seek professional help. Through therapy, Eric was able to uncover the emotional baggage he had been carrying and develop healthy coping mechanisms. With time, he regained his emotional well-being and began to feel more connected to his family and work.

Conclusion

Male depression often goes unrecognized, especially in midlife, because it doesn't fit the typical stereotype of sadness or despair. Instead, it may present as irritability, withdrawal, burnout, or even low-grade rage. These emotional states are often seen as normal reactions to life stressors, but they are often signs of deeper, unresolved emotional pain. Recognizing and understanding these symptoms is the first step toward healing.

By embracing self-awareness and seeking professional help when needed, men can address their depression in a healthy and proactive way. Depression is not a sign of weakness—it's a signal that something needs attention, and with the right tools, men can learn to manage their emotions and live healthier, more fulfilling lives.

CHAPTER 8

EMOTIONAL MAINTENANCE – DAILY HABITS THAT WORK

Introduction

In midlife, men often experience a convergence of personal and professional challenges that demand more emotional resilience and mental strength than ever before. Whether it's dealing with the pressures of career stagnation, health concerns, family dynamics, or the existential questions that arise during this stage, emotional well-being becomes a cornerstone of success and fulfillment. The truth is, emotional strength doesn't simply emerge in times of crisis; it's cultivated daily through consistent, intentional habits. Emotional maintenance, much like physical fitness, requires regular practice and attention.

In this chapter, we will explore the tools and strategies that can help men maintain emotional fitness every day. These tools— journaling, breathwork, mindfulness, and the establishment of a 15-minute daily emotional hygiene routine—are designed to be simple yet powerful ways to ground oneself emotionally. They help men develop a resilient mindset, build emotional clarity, and manage the inevitable stress and anxieties of life.

The concept of emotional maintenance goes beyond reactive self-care—it's a proactive approach to maintaining balance and focus. Through small, daily rituals, men can build a foundation of emotional strength that empowers them to navigate life's challenges with clarity and confidence.

This chapter will provide the framework for building a calm center in your life, laying out practical steps that you can incorporate into your routine. Each habit serves as a brick that, when stacked together, creates an unshakable emotional foundation.

1. Tactical Tools: Journaling, Breathwork, Mindfulness

Journaling: The Power of Writing Your Emotions

One of the simplest and most effective emotional maintenance tools is journaling. Writing down your thoughts, feelings, and reflections each day can have a transformative impact on mental well-being. Journaling serves several purposes:

- Clarity and Insight: Writing allows you to gain clarity on your emotions. Sometimes, just the act of putting thoughts on paper can help you process confusion or frustration. It brings your subconscious emotions to the surface and helps you better understand your internal world.

- Stress Release: Journaling can also serve as a release valve for pent-up emotions. Whether it's stress from work, family, or personal life, writing gives you an outlet to express feelings that you might otherwise bottle up. Instead of internalizing frustration or resentment, you externalize it onto the page.

- Goal-Setting and Reflection: Regular journaling can help you stay focused on your goals, track progress, and reflect on your personal growth. It serves as both a tool for reflection and a way to set intentions for the day, week, or month.

How to Start Journaling:

- Morning Pages: One of the most effective journaling practices is Morning Pages, a concept made popular by author Julia Cameron in her book *The Artist's Way*. This practice involves writing three pages of stream-of-consciousness thoughts first thing in the morning. The goal is not to structure the writing or filter the content, but to let the mind unload. It clears mental clutter and makes space for focus and creativity.

- Prompt-Based Journaling: If Morning Pages feels too overwhelming, start with a few guiding prompts. For example:

    o What am I feeling right now?

    o What am I grateful for today?

    o What is my biggest challenge right now, and how can I address it?

Real-life Example:

- John, a 45-year-old teacher, found that journaling helped him manage the increasing stress he felt as his career progressed. He started writing each morning before school to clear his mind. Over time, he found that journaling not only helped him de-stress but also gave him clarity on his personal goals and work-life balance. His relationship with his spouse improved as well, as journaling gave him the emotional outlet he needed to process his feelings and communicate more openly.

Breathwork: The Power of the Breath to Reset Your Nervous System

Breathing is one of the most powerful tools available for emotional regulation. Breathwork involves conscious, controlled breathing techniques designed to activate the parasympathetic nervous system (the "rest and digest" system), which calms the body and mind. Breathwork is incredibly effective for reducing stress, anxiety, and the physical symptoms of emotional strain.

- Deep Breathing: Deep diaphragmatic breathing is one of the most basic yet effective forms of breathwork. This type of breathing encourages the full expansion of the lungs, stimulating the body's relaxation response.

- Box Breathing: Box breathing, also known as square breathing, is a simple yet effective technique. It involves breathing in for a count of four, holding the breath for four, exhaling for four, and holding again for four. This technique helps to reduce anxiety and increase focus.

- The 4-7-8 Method: Another effective method is the 4-7-8 breathing technique. Inhale for a count of four, hold the breath for seven, and then exhale for eight. This pattern is particularly helpful for calming the nervous system and promoting relaxation.

How to Practice Breathwork:

- Start with 5 minutes a day: Set aside time each day to practice deep breathing. Whether you do it in the morning, during lunch, or before bed, consistent practice can have a profound impact on your ability to manage stress.

- Incorporate breathwork during stressful moments: Whenever you feel overwhelmed, anxious, or tense, take a few minutes to practice controlled breathing. Focus entirely on the sensation of the breath moving in and out of your body. This can serve as a quick reset during high-stress situations.

Real-life Example:

- Andrew, a 48-year-old marketing executive, often found himself feeling anxious before important meetings. He used to feel his heart racing and his mind becoming overwhelmed with stress. By learning breathwork techniques, Andrew could manage his anxiety before meetings. Using box breathing in the moments leading up to a presentation helped him stay calm, centered, and present.

2. 15-Minute Emotional Hygiene Routine for Mental Strength

Emotional hygiene is the practice of maintaining your emotional health in the same way you would maintain physical hygiene. Just as brushing your teeth and washing your face are essential parts of daily life, engaging in regular emotional hygiene can improve your overall well-being. A 15-minute emotional hygiene routine can help men clear mental clutter, process emotions, and build resilience against the stressors of the day.

The 15-Minute Routine Breakdown:

1. Mindfulness Moment (5 minutes):

- Find a quiet space where you can sit comfortably. Focus on your breath, noticing each inhalation and exhalation. Mindfulness meditation allows you to become aware of your thoughts and emotions without judgment, creating a space for clarity and emotional balance.

2. Journaling (5 minutes):

- After your mindfulness moment, spend five minutes writing. It could be about your current emotional state, thoughts on the day ahead, or anything that has been bothering you. This brief writing session helps to offload emotions and gain perspective.

3. Breathwork (5 minutes):

- Finish the routine with breathwork. You can use box breathing or the 4-7-8 method to center yourself. This will not only calm your nervous system but also give you a sense of control over your emotional state.

Real-life Example:

- Brad, a 50-year-old father and entrepreneur, was juggling the demands of his business with family responsibilities. He found that taking just 15 minutes each morning for his emotional hygiene routine made a huge difference in his emotional clarity throughout the day. By integrating mindfulness, journaling, and breathwork into his routine, he was better equipped to handle stress, make clear decisions, and communicate effectively with his team and family.

3. Building a Calm Center, One Brick at a Time

Emotional fitness, like physical fitness, is built over time through consistent practice. The goal is not to completely eliminate stress or emotions but to develop the resilience needed to manage them effectively. Think of emotional fitness as building a strong, unshakable center within yourself, where you can remain grounded even during turbulent moments.

Each emotional hygiene practice is like a brick in the foundation of your calm center. When you commit to these daily habits—whether it's journaling, breathwork, or mindfulness— you're building a sense of stability that will help you navigate life's inevitable ups and downs.

The process of building this calm center doesn't happen overnight. It requires patience, persistence, and consistency. Just as muscles grow stronger with regular exercise, your emotional muscles grow stronger when you practice emotional fitness daily. Over time, you will develop a more resilient emotional core, which will allow you to stay centered, focused, and emotionally balanced in even the most challenging circumstances.

Real-life Example:

- Ethan, a 44-year-old project manager, began implementing daily emotional hygiene practices after he realized he was becoming increasingly stressed and irritable at work. He committed to a 15-minute routine each morning and found that, over time, he was more present and effective in his personal and professional life. His relationships improved, and he felt more mentally clear and emotionally balanced throughout the day.

Conclusion

The emotional challenges that come with midlife—stress, burnout, anxiety—are part of the human experience. However, managing these challenges doesn't require superhuman strength or emotional repression; it requires consistent emotional maintenance. By embracing daily habits such as journaling, breathwork, and mindfulness, men can develop the emotional resilience needed to navigate the ups and downs of life with confidence and clarity.

The 15-minute emotional hygiene routine serves as a simple yet powerful practice that can be incorporated into any busy schedule. These small, consistent actions—when practiced every day—will build the foundation of emotional fitness that every man needs to maintain mental strength, emotional balance, and overall well-being. By building a calm center one brick at a time, men can create a life of emotional stability, inner peace, and resilience, making midlife not a crisis, but a period of growth, reflection, and self-empowerment.

CHAPTER 9

BROTHER, NOT ALONE – FINDING YOUR CIRCLE

Introduction

As men approach their 40s, the demands of work, family, and personal health often consume their time and emotional energy. While friendships are a vital aspect of human well-being, many men find that their social circles become smaller or more distant as they age. The transition from youthful camaraderie to the responsibilities of adulthood can leave men feeling isolated or disconnected, even when surrounded by people. At midlife, many men look around and realize that they no longer have the same close friendships they once did, and some may not have any close male friends at all.

In a world that often encourages men to be self-reliant and avoid emotional vulnerability, the importance of male friendships cannot be overstated. Male friendships are not just about shared activities like sports or banter—they provide the emotional support, validation, and companionship that are essential for mental well-being. Yet, for many men, the idea of fostering deeper, more authentic connections with other men feels foreign, even awkward. This chapter seeks to explore the significance of male friendships in midlife, why these relationships often fade after 40, and how to create meaningful connections with other men that go beyond surface-level interactions.

We'll dive into the reasons why male friendships tend to fade over time, how to build authentic and supportive relationships beyond banter and shared activities, and how to embrace vulnerability without feeling uncomfortable or "cringe." By the end of this chapter, you'll understand the vital role male friendships play in midlife and how you can cultivate a brotherhood that provides both emotional support and a sense of belonging.

1. The Importance of Male Friendships (and Why They Fade After 40)

Friendships are an essential aspect of human life, and they are no less important for men as they age. However, research consistently shows that men tend to have fewer close friends as they move into midlife, with many reporting social isolation or loneliness. The phenomenon of shrinking social circles in midlife is not just a passing phase; it's a reflection of changing priorities, evolving personal dynamics, and shifting societal expectations.

Why Male Friendships Fade Over Time

As men reach their 40s, their priorities shift. The demands of work, the pressure to provide for their families, and the physical and emotional toll of aging often take precedence over socializing. There are several factors contributing to the fading of male friendships after 40:

1. Increased Family and Work Obligations: At midlife, many men are deeply entrenched in family life and career. The responsibilities of raising children, caring for aging parents, and maintaining demanding work schedules often

leave little time for social activities. In the past, socializing with friends may have been spontaneous and frequent, but now, it requires intentional effort. Without time for casual hangouts or shared experiences, friendships can wither.

2. Changing Interests and Priorities: As men grow older, their interests may evolve. Where once there was a strong emphasis on shared hobbies or physical activities, those interests may change or become less frequent. The bonds formed through activities like playing sports or drinking with friends may not hold the same appeal as they once did. When shared interests fade, it becomes harder to sustain friendships based solely on those activities.

3. Emotional Distance and Vulnerability: Men are often socialized to view vulnerability as a weakness. As a result, they may struggle to form deep emotional connections with their male friends. While shared laughter and banter are often the glue that holds male friendships together, these interactions rarely provide the depth needed to support men through the challenges of midlife. Over time, without emotional intimacy, friendships may become shallow and distant.

4. Fear of Judgment or Awkwardness: As men age, they may feel more self-conscious about expressing vulnerability or discussing emotions with friends. They may fear judgment or ridicule, leading them to retreat emotionally. The idea of opening up to friends about personal struggles, whether related to mental health, relationships, or career frustrations, can seem uncomfortable or even embarrassing.

The Cost of Friendship Loss in Midlife

The loss of close male friendships can have a profound impact on a man's well-being. Male friendships are not just for companionship—they are essential for emotional and psychological health. Studies show that men who have strong social connections live longer, healthier, and happier lives. The absence of male friendships can contribute to feelings of loneliness, stress, and emotional distress.

- Social Isolation and Mental Health: The absence of a supportive social network can increase the risk of mental health issues such as depression, anxiety, and stress. Without friends to turn to for emotional support or guidance, men may find it harder to manage the stresses of midlife.

- Lack of Emotional Outlet: Men are often taught to internalize their emotions, leading to a lack of emotional outlets. Healthy friendships offer a safe space to express feelings, whether it's discussing career frustrations, health concerns, or family issues. When men lack these emotional outlets, they may resort to unhealthy coping mechanisms like substance abuse, anger, or withdrawal.

Real-life Example:

- James, a 47-year-old business owner, found himself feeling increasingly isolated after his friends drifted away. As his work became more demanding and his family obligations grew, he stopped seeing his friends. He missed the camaraderie and shared experiences they once had, but he didn't know how to reconnect. Over time, James noticed that his stress levels increased, and he began feeling more anxious and irritable. It wasn't until he started reaching out to old friends that he realized how much he had been missing the emotional support and connection that male friendships provide.

2. How to Build Authentic Connections Beyond Banter and Sports

While shared activities like sports or drinking are often the foundation of many male friendships, they don't provide the emotional depth needed to sustain meaningful connections over time. To build authentic male friendships, men must move beyond surface-level interactions and create opportunities for emotional intimacy and support. This doesn't mean abandoning traditional male bonding activities like watching sports, but it does involve adding a layer of vulnerability and authenticity to those interactions.

Key Steps to Building Authentic Friendships

1. Start with Intentionality: To build stronger male friendships, you must make the effort to prioritize them. Reach out to old friends, invite them for regular meetups, and actively create opportunities for meaningful conversations. Friendships, like all relationships, require effort to maintain.

2. Embrace Vulnerability: Authentic connections are built on vulnerability. This doesn't mean sharing every detail of your life, but it does involve being open about your challenges, struggles, and emotions. Don't wait for a crisis to open up—create the space for honest conversations in everyday interactions.

- Example: Instead of talking only about sports scores or work achievements, ask a friend, "How are you really doing?" or share something personal, such as a struggle you're facing at work or with your health. This can lead to deeper conversations and help you build a more authentic connection.

3. Show Up Consistently: Authentic friendships are built on trust and consistency. Show up for your friends, both in good times and bad. This means being present at significant moments in their lives—whether it's a birthday, a family event, or a time of crisis. It also means checking in regularly, even if it's just a text or a quick call.

4. Embrace Growth Together: As men grow older, their priorities shift, and so do their friendships. Embrace the opportunity to grow with your friends. Engage in activities that promote personal growth and self-awareness, such as attending workshops, joining a fitness group, or even doing community service together. Growing together can deepen your bond and create a sense of shared purpose.

Real-life Example:

▪ Michael, a 46-year-old executive, realized that his friendships had become shallow, primarily revolving around occasional drinks or watching games. He made a conscious decision to take his friendships to a deeper level. He began to reach out to a few close friends with more meaningful questions like, "What's the hardest part of your life right now?" or "How do you deal with stress?" This change in his approach led to more emotionally fulfilling conversations and strengthened his friendships over time.

3. Vulnerability in Male Circles Without the Cringe

While vulnerability is essential for authentic connections, many men still view it as uncomfortable or even "cringe-worthy." The idea of sharing personal feelings or struggles with other men can seem foreign or awkward, especially in a society that has long encouraged men to be stoic, self-sufficient, and emotionally reserved. However, vulnerability is not a weakness; it is the very foundation of emotional strength and resilience.

Overcoming the "Cringe" Factor

1. Normalize Vulnerability: Start small and normalize vulnerability in your interactions. Sharing your own feelings, no matter how minor, can help break down barriers and make emotional expression feel more natural. It's about creating a safe space where everyone can be open without fear of judgment.

2. Lead by Example: If you want your friends to open up, you have to be the first to lead by example. Share your own struggles, fears, or challenges, and you'll find that others will follow suit. Vulnerability often inspires vulnerability, and it's through mutual openness that connections are deepened.

3. Create a Safe Environment: In male circles, it's important to create a culture of respect and acceptance. If a friend shares something vulnerable, avoid making jokes, dismissing feelings, or offering unsolicited advice. Instead, listen actively and offer empathy and support.

Real-life Example:

- Ryan, a 49-year-old lawyer, had always kept his emotions to himself, believing that sharing personal struggles would make him appear weak. However, after a tough period at work, Ryan started opening up to a close friend. He shared his frustrations and fears about his career and personal life. To his surprise, his friend responded with empathy and shared similar experiences. This moment of vulnerability deepened their bond, leading to a more supportive and meaningful friendship.

Conclusion

The importance of male friendships in midlife cannot be overstated. As men approach their 40s, the need for emotional connection, support, and authenticity in friendships becomes more critical than ever. By building connections that go beyond banter and surface-level interactions, men can create a circle of brothers who offer emotional support, understanding, and accountability.

Vulnerability, once seen as uncomfortable or "cringe," is a vital tool for building deeper, more meaningful relationships. By embracing vulnerability, practicing empathy, and creating a safe space for emotional expression, men can forge stronger connections and experience greater mental well-being. The friendships you cultivate in midlife will provide not only support and companionship but also a sense of belonging and purpose that enriches your emotional life.

CHAPTER 10

MIDLIFE TRANSITIONS – CAREER, PURPOSE, IDENTITY

Introduction: The Crossroads of Midlife

Midlife is often described as a crossroads—a time when life slows down, but also speeds up in new, unexpected ways. By the time men reach their 40s, they've likely accomplished much: they've built careers, established families, and reached a certain level of professional or personal success. But something changes. The dreams and ambitions that once felt so vibrant and clear may now feel empty or unfulfilled. Men might feel as though they've plateaued in their careers, or they may be questioning whether the goals they've been pursuing are still relevant to their evolving sense of self.

It's easy to assume that the midlife crisis is a phenomenon reserved for a small minority of people, but the reality is that many men experience some form of existential questioning or self-doubt during this phase of life. The transition that occurs in midlife is not just about the external changes (e.g., aging, career shifts, family dynamics); it's about the internal shift in identity and purpose.

In this chapter, we will explore three core areas that men often face during midlife transitions:

1. Career Plateau and Reinvention: After years of striving and climbing, many men find themselves at a plateau. Success

feels empty, and the drive for more seems less meaningful. This section will explore the common experiences of career stagnation, the desire for reinvention, and how men can navigate these crossroads.

2. Letting Go of Outdated Dreams and Redefining Meaning: The dreams and values that once shaped a man's life may no longer fit as he matures. This section will dive into the process of letting go of outdated dreams and the importance of redefining what truly matters in this stage of life.

3. You Are Not Your Job – You're Your Values: Midlife offers the opportunity to disconnect self-worth from career achievements. Many men in midlife tie their sense of identity to their job or professional success, but true fulfillment comes from aligning life with personal values. This section will provide a framework for exploring identity beyond the career and building a life based on deeper, more enduring principles.

Through this exploration, men will learn how to embrace midlife as a time of renewal, redefinition, and purposeful reinvention, rather than a crisis.

1. When Success Feels Empty: Career Plateau and Reinvention

The Midlife Career Plateau: The Paradox of Success

By the time men reach their 40s, they've typically achieved a certain level of success in their careers. Whether that success is defined by job title, financial stability, or professional accolades, many men in midlife experience a career plateau—a sense that they've hit a ceiling and that their efforts are no longer yielding the same excitement or rewards they once did.

For some men, the experience of career success can feel somewhat empty. The very achievements that they once aspired to—promotions, recognition, or financial milestones—no longer provide the satisfaction they thought they would. They may feel like they've "done it all," but now, those external achievements fail to offer the same sense of fulfillment.

- Symptoms of the Career Plateau: The most common symptoms of career stagnation include lack of enthusiasm for daily tasks, feelings of disconnection from the work, and frustration with limited growth opportunities. What was once exciting and challenging now feels monotonous and uninspiring. Some men may even experience a sense of regret about the career path they chose years ago.

- The Internal Conflict: Despite the external markers of success, many men in midlife feel an internal conflict—a yearning for something more meaningful or aligned with their evolving sense of self. There may be a desire to reinvent themselves, but uncertainty about how to proceed can hold them back. They may feel stuck, torn between the desire for change and the comfort of the familiar.

The Desire for Reinvention

The desire for career reinvention is a natural part of the midlife process. As men reassess their goals and values, they may feel drawn to redefine their professional identity. The desire for reinvention can be both liberating and intimidating. It requires courage to step away from a path that has provided stability, and it demands vulnerability to acknowledge the possibility of failure or uncertainty.

- Career Transitions and Shifts: Reinventing oneself professionally doesn't necessarily mean quitting a job or changing careers entirely. It could involve seeking out new responsibilities, taking on different challenges, or finding new ways to approach one's current role. Many men in midlife opt for career transition—moving from one area of expertise to another—or they explore opportunities for entrepreneurship or consulting.

- The Pursuit of Passion: In midlife, many men realize that their passion or purpose no longer aligns with the corporate grind or the career they once thought was the right path. Some may seek careers that allow them to express their creative talents or pursue causes they care about. This can be a powerful catalyst for reinvention, as it involves aligning work with meaningful values.

Real-life Example:

- Tom, a 48-year-old lawyer, had spent 20 years in a corporate law firm. Although he had achieved significant success, he realized that the work no longer brought him the same sense of fulfillment it once did. He felt disconnected from the corporate world and began to explore new career paths that involved helping others. Tom decided to pivot to a career in non-profit work, where he could leverage his legal expertise to advocate for social justice. The transition wasn't easy, but it brought him a renewed sense of purpose.

Facing Fear of Change: The Emotional Process of Reinvention

Reinvention requires men to face their fears and uncertainty. The fear of the unknown, of failure, or of giving up the security of a long-established career, can be overwhelming. Men may worry about losing their identity or status when they move away from a role that has defined them for years.

However, embracing change is often the key to unlocking new opportunities. Reinvention is an act of courage, one that involves confronting self-doubt and embracing the possibility of growth and renewal.

2. Letting Go of Outdated Dreams and Redefining Meaning

As men enter midlife, they often realize that the dreams and ambitions they held in their youth are no longer in alignment with their current values. The goals that once felt essential—whether related to career, family, or personal achievements—may no longer feel relevant. Letting go of outdated dreams is one of the most liberating steps a man can take toward living an authentic life.

Why Outdated Dreams Hold Us Back

Outdated dreams can trap men in false narratives about who they are and what they should be achieving. Many men grow up with a set of expectations about success: get a good job, earn a steady income, climb the career ladder, and provide for their family. While these are admirable goals, they don't necessarily align with the deeper, more personal meaning men seek as they grow older.

- The Cost of Clinging to Old Dreams: Holding onto outdated dreams can prevent men from embracing new possibilities. They may continue to chase after achievements or milestones that no longer bring them joy or fulfillment. This can result in feelings of frustration, dissatisfaction, and burnout.

- Reevaluating Priorities: Midlife provides an opportunity to reevaluate priorities and consider what is truly important. For some, this means letting go of career-based aspirations in favor of personal growth, well-being, or family time. It may involve redefining what success means and pursuing a path that is more aligned with current passions, values, and needs.

Redefining Meaning: Creating a New Vision

Letting go of outdated dreams does not mean giving up on the desire for success or fulfillment—it means creating a new vision of what those concepts mean. Midlife is an opportunity to redefine meaning and build a future that resonates with personal values.

- Living with Purpose: The key to finding new meaning is understanding that life is not just about external achievement but about living with purpose. Whether that purpose is rooted in family, personal growth, contribution, or creativity, it's about pursuing what feels most authentic.

- Aligning Goals with Values: Redefining meaning requires aligning your goals with your core values. Men in midlife may find that their values have shifted—what was once important may no longer hold the same weight. By identifying what truly matters, men can create a new roadmap for the second half of their lives.

Real-life Example:

- Dave, a 50-year-old entrepreneur, spent his entire career focused on building his business empire. However, after a health scare, Dave realized that his professional success had come at the expense of his health, relationships, and well-being. He decided to let go of his long-standing dream of expanding his business and instead focused on creating a balanced lifestyle that included time for family, fitness, and travel. This shift brought him greater happiness and a more sustainable sense of success.

3. You Are Not Your Job – You're Your Values

One of the most significant realizations that men have in midlife is that their identity is not tied to their job or career. For many men, their job has been the central pillar of their self-worth for decades. But when that job no longer provides the same satisfaction, or when it feels empty, it's easy to become lost or confused.

Disconnecting Self-Worth from Career

As men approach midlife, they must confront the fact that self-worth should not be tied exclusively to professional achievements. Midlife is a time to redefine what it means to be successful and fulfilled. A man's value is not solely determined by his career status, income, or title—it's determined by his values, his relationships, and his actions.

- The Challenge of Identity Crisis: Men in midlife may experience an identity crisis if they've defined themselves primarily by their job or role. When that job is no longer fulfilling or when they're faced with professional setbacks, they may feel like they've lost their sense of purpose. Reframing identity to include a broader sense of self-worth beyond career achievements is crucial to overcoming this crisis.

- Defining Values and Priorities: Midlife offers an opportunity to identify and define the values that truly matter. These may include family, personal growth, community, creativity, or contribution. Once a man understands his core values, he can start aligning his actions with those values, creating a deeper sense of purpose.

Real-life Example:

- Robert, a 52-year-old architect, spent most of his career building a successful firm. However, after a series of personal losses and a growing sense of dissatisfaction, Robert began questioning his life's direction. He realized that his identity had been too intertwined with his profession. By shifting his focus to his personal values—family, health, and creativity—he was able to redefine his purpose. He gradually shifted from a demanding career to mentoring younger architects and dedicating time to his family and personal projects.

Conclusion

Midlife is a pivotal time in a man's life, marked by self-reflection, reassessment, and growth. The transition from the career-driven, achievement-oriented self to a more purpose-driven and values-oriented life can be challenging but ultimately liberating. By recognizing the empty feeling that may accompany career success, letting go of outdated dreams, and shifting focus to personal values, men can redefine their sense of identity and meaning.

Midlife is not the end of growth—it is the beginning of a new chapter. By embracing the process of reinvention, letting go of past limitations, and prioritizing authentic fulfillment, men can create a richer, more meaningful life. Midlife offers a unique opportunity to build a future that is deeply aligned with who you are at this stage of life, not who you were decades ago.

PHYSICAL STRENGTH, MENTAL RESILIENCE

Introduction: The Power of the Body-Mind Connection

As men reach their 40s, their physical health can significantly impact their emotional and mental well-being. The physical challenges of aging—such as decreasing testosterone levels, muscle mass, energy levels, and mobility—often seem to occur simultaneously with the emotional and psychological shifts of midlife. However, maintaining physical health at this stage of life is not just about aesthetics or strength; it's deeply linked to mental resilience.

In fact, the brain-body connection is one of the most powerful yet overlooked relationships in mental health. Movement, exercise, and maintaining an active lifestyle do more than just improve the body—they have a direct impact on the brain, influencing mood, mental clarity, and overall emotional regulation. Physical activity plays a key role in maintaining testosterone levels, reducing stress, and enhancing mental clarity, while also boosting vitality, sleep, and sex drive.

This chapter will explore how maintaining physical strength supports mental resilience in men over 40, examining the intersection of fitness, testosterone, and emotional well-being. It will also provide insights into effective fitness routines for mental clarity and discuss how sleep, sex drive, and vitality are all deeply connected to physical health as men age.

1. The Brain-Body Connection: Movement, Testosterone, and Mood

How Physical Activity Affects Mental Health

There is no doubt that regular physical activity has a profound effect on mental health. But the link between movement and mood is often underestimated. The body's physical systems and mental processes are inextricably connected, and the act of engaging in regular movement not only improves cardiovascular health, muscle strength, and flexibility, but it also boosts cognitive function and mood.

The Impact of Exercise on the Brain

- Endorphin Release: Exercise triggers the release of endorphins, the body's natural "feel-good" chemicals, which can help combat feelings of stress, anxiety, and depression. Endorphins are often referred to as the body's natural painkillers, and their release during exercise promotes positive feelings and can help fight off negative emotions like frustration and sadness.

- Neuroplasticity: Physical activity, especially aerobic exercise, enhances neuroplasticity—the brain's ability to adapt and reorganize itself. This means that movement not only improves physical well-being but also strengthens cognitive function. It improves focus, memory, and learning abilities, which can be especially valuable during midlife when mental sharpness is a priority.

- Stress Reduction: Exercise also helps regulate the HPA (hypothalamic-pituitary-adrenal) axis, the part of the body responsible for stress responses. Regular exercise reduces the levels of cortisol (the stress hormone) and adrenaline, both of which can contribute to feelings of anxiety, agitation, or burnout.

Real-life Example:

- Michael, a 46-year-old teacher, had been feeling overwhelmed with work and family life. His energy levels were low, and he often felt irritable and disconnected. After a couple of months of regular aerobic exercise—like cycling and swimming—Michael began to notice significant improvements. He felt calmer, more focused, and his stress levels decreased. His newfound energy boosted his confidence and allowed him to be more present with his family and colleagues.

Testosterone: A Key Player in Mental and Physical Health

Testosterone, often referred to as the "male hormone," plays a crucial role in both physical and mental health, especially as men age. Testosterone is responsible for muscle growth, bone density, energy levels, and libido. It also impacts mood, cognitive function, and emotional regulation. As men approach 40 and beyond, their testosterone levels naturally begin to decline, which can contribute to feelings of fatigue, depression, irritability, and decreased motivation.

- Exercise, particularly strength training and high-intensity interval training (HIIT), can help maintain and even increase testosterone production. This is crucial for maintaining both physical strength and mental resilience.

- Strength Training and Testosterone: Engaging in resistance training, such as lifting weights or bodyweight exercises, stimulates the production of testosterone and helps to counteract its natural decline. Research shows that regular strength training can lead to an increase in free testosterone levels, which are essential for mood regulation, motivation, and energy levels.

- HIIT for Testosterone: High-intensity interval training (HIIT) is another exercise modality that has been shown to increase testosterone levels. HIIT involves alternating between intense bursts of activity and short recovery periods. This type of workout not only boosts cardiovascular health but also promotes hormonal balance, including the production of testosterone.

Real-life Example:

- David, a 50-year-old accountant, noticed a decline in his energy and motivation after he turned 45. He felt sluggish and lacked the energy he once had. After starting a strength training routine three times a week, he noticed a marked improvement in both his physical strength and mood. His energy levels were higher, he felt more motivated, and his mental clarity significantly improved. David's experience illustrates how regular strength training can positively impact testosterone production and mental resilience.

2. Fitness Routines for Mental Clarity

As men age, they may experience a decline in mental clarity or cognitive function. However, staying physically active can counteract this decline and promote sharper cognitive function. Certain types of physical activities are particularly beneficial for enhancing mental clarity and focus.

Aerobic Exercise for Cognitive Health

Aerobic exercises, such as running, cycling, and swimming, have been shown to improve cognitive function by increasing blood flow to the brain and promoting the growth of new brain cells. Regular aerobic exercise can improve memory, focus, and mental sharpness, helping men remain mentally agile as they age.

- Improved Blood Flow: Aerobic exercise increases blood flow to the brain, which helps nourish brain cells and improve oxygen delivery. This supports enhanced mental clarity, greater concentration, and better cognitive function overall.

- Cognitive Benefits: Studies show that regular aerobic exercise can improve memory and attention span by stimulating the hippocampus, the part of the brain associated with learning and memory. This can be particularly beneficial for men in midlife who may experience a decline in memory or mental focus.

Real-life Example:

- Gary, a 47-year-old engineer, struggled with brain fog and difficulty focusing at work. He began incorporating a daily 30-minute jog into his routine. Over the course of a few weeks, Gary noticed that his mental clarity improved significantly. He felt more focused during meetings and had an easier time managing tasks at work.

Strength Training for Mental Toughness

Strength training doesn't just improve physical strength—it also enhances mental toughness. The act of pushing your body to lift heavier weights, complete more reps, or perform more challenging exercises can help build resilience and mental endurance. Strength training requires focus and discipline, both of which can help improve cognitive function and boost overall mental clarity.

- Building Discipline and Focus: Strength training is one of the most effective ways to develop mental resilience. It requires consistent effort, dedication, and the ability to push through discomfort—all of which translate into improved mental toughness in other areas of life.

- Boosting Confidence and Mental Health: Strength training can improve confidence by creating a tangible sense of achievement. Every time a person lifts more weight, completes more reps, or makes progress, they reinforce the connection between physical effort and mental strength.

Real-life Example:

- Tony, a 45-year-old teacher, used to struggle with low self-esteem and mental fatigue. After joining a local gym and committing to strength training, Tony noticed significant changes in his mindset. As he built strength, he felt more empowered, which carried over into his personal life and work. He reported feeling more mentally sharp and better able to handle stress.

3. Sleep, Sex Drive, and Vitality After 40

Sleep: The Foundation of Mental and Physical Health

As men age, sleep patterns tend to change, and poor sleep quality can have a significant impact on mental clarity, emotional regulation, and overall well-being. Sleep is the foundation of health—it affects everything from cognitive function to stress management to testosterone production.

- The Importance of Sleep: Sleep is when the body and mind repair themselves. During deep sleep, the body restores energy, consolidates memories, and performs vital functions like hormone production. For men over 40, ensuring they get sufficient and quality sleep is crucial for maintaining mental clarity, emotional stability, and testosterone levels.

- Sleep Deprivation and Its Impact: Sleep deprivation can increase levels of cortisol (the stress hormone) and decrease testosterone levels. It can lead to mental fog, irritability, and increased stress levels. Prioritizing good sleep hygiene is essential for both physical and emotional well-being.

Sex Drive: Testosterone and Vitality

Testosterone plays a major role in sexual health and libido. As men age, testosterone naturally declines, which can impact sex drive and overall vitality. However, maintaining an active lifestyle—particularly through strength training and aerobic exercise—can help mitigate the decline in testosterone and improve sexual health.

- Exercise and Sex Drive: Regular physical activity, particularly strength training and HIIT, can boost testosterone levels, which in turn supports healthy libido and sexual performance. Physical fitness also increases circulation, which contributes to better sexual health and vitality.

- Testosterone and Vitality: Testosterone is not only important for sexual health—it also affects energy levels, mood, and motivation. Keeping testosterone levels balanced through exercise and a healthy lifestyle can help men feel more energetic, focused, and motivated.

Real-life Example:

- Rick, a 48-year-old architect, had noticed a decline in his libido and energy levels over the past few years. After incorporating a strength training routine and improving his sleep habits, Rick noticed a significant improvement in his sex drive and overall vitality. His relationships improved, and he felt more confident and energized.

Conclusion

Midlife is a time of transition, and maintaining both physical strength and mental resilience is crucial for navigating this period with vitality and purpose. The brain-body connection is powerful—regular exercise and physical activity have profound effects on mental clarity, mood regulation, and emotional well-being. By incorporating strength training, aerobic exercise, and other fitness routines into daily life, men can boost testosterone, enhance cognitive function, and build emotional resilience. Additionally, prioritizing sleep and managing stress are key components of maintaining vitality and overall health.

Through these practices, men can not only improve their physical strength but also nurture their mental resilience, allowing them to thrive in midlife and beyond.

THE MIND-BODY DISCONNECT – WHAT YOUR BODY'S TRYING TO TELL YOU

Introduction: The Body Speaks, But Are We Listening?

In our fast-paced, achievement-oriented culture, it's easy to ignore the signals our bodies send us. Men, in particular, often face societal pressure to be strong, resilient, and unaffected by their emotions, leading many to disconnect from the more subtle messages their bodies are trying to convey. We often treat physical symptoms as isolated events or inconveniences—headaches, back pain, fatigue, digestive issues—without considering that they may be the body's way of communicating deeper emotional or psychological distress.

This chapter explores the often-overlooked connection between the body and mind, shedding light on how physical symptoms can be emotional cues and why it's crucial to pay attention to these signals. As men age, particularly in their 40s and beyond, the cumulative effects of chronic stress, poor gut health, inflammation, and unresolved emotional issues may manifest in physical forms. The body's response to emotional turmoil, stress, or unresolved trauma often leads to a disconnect that can have profound effects on both mental and physical health.

We will dive deep into the science behind this connection and how chronic stress, poor gut health, and inflammation can impact mood, mental clarity, and overall well-being. This chapter will also discuss the hidden costs of ignoring these physical symptoms and offer strategies to reconnect the mind and body for better health and emotional balance.

1. Listening to Physical Symptoms as Emotional Cues

The mind and body are intricately connected, and often, what is happening in one part of the body is directly linked to an emotional state or psychological process. However, in many cases, these signals go unnoticed or unaddressed.

The Body as a Messenger

Physical symptoms such as muscle tension, fatigue, headaches, and digestive issues can be directly related to emotional stress. These symptoms are the body's way of signaling that something is wrong emotionally or psychologically. Instead of simply masking these symptoms with medications or quick fixes, it's important to listen and interpret them as clues to what may be happening beneath the surface.

- Muscle Tension and Tightness: One of the most common physical manifestations of emotional stress is muscle tension. Men, especially in midlife, may carry the weight of their responsibilities—work, family, health—directly in their shoulders, neck, and back. This tension often represents the emotional burden they carry, manifesting as tightness, pain, or discomfort.

- Fatigue and Lack of Energy: Chronic fatigue is often more than just a result of poor sleep or overwork. It's a signal that the body is under emotional duress. Men who suppress emotions or who are constantly "on the go" may find themselves feeling mentally and physically exhausted, even after a full night's sleep.

- Headaches and Migraines: The frequent occurrence of headaches, particularly tension headaches or migraines, can indicate that there are unaddressed stressors or unresolved emotional tension. These headaches are often related to the mind's inability to process or release built-up emotional pressure.

- Digestive Issues: Gut health is intrinsically linked to emotional well-being. The gut is often referred to as the "second brain," due to its connection to the central nervous system. Emotional distress, anxiety, or unresolved grief can disrupt digestion, leading to issues like irritable bowel syndrome (IBS), bloating, constipation, and diarrhea. When we experience stress, the digestive system is one of the first areas to react.

Real-life Example:

- John, a 44-year-old manager, was experiencing frequent back pain and tension in his neck. After months of seeing physical therapists without significant improvement, he realized that his pain wasn't solely physical—it was connected to the constant stress he was under at work and at home. His emotional distress was manifesting physically in the form of muscle tension. Once he started addressing his emotional stress through therapy and regular physical activity, his pain significantly decreased, illustrating how emotional factors can manifest physically.

Chronic Stress and Its Impact on the Body

Chronic stress, particularly unacknowledged or unmanaged emotional stress, is a powerful force that affects the body in profound ways. Cortisol, the body's primary stress hormone, is essential for handling short bursts of stress, but prolonged or chronic exposure to cortisol can have damaging effects on physical health, mood, and mental clarity.

- Increased Muscle Tension: Prolonged stress leads to increased muscle tension, making it more difficult to relax physically. The body becomes stuck in a constant state of fight-or-flight, leading to persistent neck pain, back pain, and muscle soreness. This tension can also disrupt sleep, creating a cycle of stress and physical discomfort.

- Immune System Suppression: Chronic stress also weakens the immune system, making the body more vulnerable to illnesses and infections. When the body is under stress for prolonged periods, it struggles to defend against pathogens and heal itself properly.

- Sleep Disturbances: Stress and anxiety can make it difficult to fall asleep, stay asleep, or achieve deep, restorative sleep. This lack of sleep can, in turn, worsen stress, creating a vicious cycle of physical and mental fatigue.

- Heart Health and Blood Pressure: Chronic stress has been linked to high blood pressure and an increased risk of cardiovascular disease. Stress increases the heart rate and constricts blood vessels, which over time can put strain on the heart.

Real-life Example:

- David, a 48-year-old lawyer, had been feeling burnt out at work for months. He noticed a sharp increase in his blood pressure, frequent headaches, and muscle pain in his shoulders and neck. Despite visiting doctors for his symptoms, nothing seemed to help. It wasn't until he addressed his stress levels and took a step back from the relentless pace of his work life that his physical symptoms began to subside. David realized that his chronic stress was physically manifesting in multiple ways, and once he implemented strategies for emotional and physical relaxation, his overall health improved significantly.

2. Gut Health, Inflammation, and Mood

The gut-brain connection has gained significant attention in recent years, particularly in relation to its impact on mood disorders, anxiety, and depression. The gut, often referred to as the body's "second brain," contains over 100 million nerve cells and is responsible for producing more than 90% of the body's serotonin, the neurotransmitter responsible for regulating mood, sleep, and digestion.

When the gut is unhealthy or imbalanced, it can have far-reaching effects on mental health. Chronic inflammation, gut dysbiosis (an imbalance of gut bacteria), and poor digestion can all lead to feelings of anxiety, irritability, fatigue, and low mood.

The Link Between Gut Health and Mental Health

- Inflammation and Depression: Chronic inflammation in the body has been linked to depression and mood disorders. Studies have shown that people with elevated levels of inflammation often experience higher rates of depression, and this inflammation can be exacerbated by poor diet, stress, and lack of physical activity.

- Gut Dysbiosis: An imbalance in gut bacteria, known as gut dysbiosis, can affect the body's ability to produce serotonin and regulate emotions. Diets high in processed foods and low in fiber can contribute to gut dysbiosis, leading to mood swings, irritability, and mental fog.

- The Impact of Stress on the Gut: Stress directly impacts the gut by increasing intestinal permeability (commonly known as "leaky gut"), which allows harmful substances to pass through the gut lining into the bloodstream, causing inflammation and immune system responses. This process can contribute to conditions like IBS, chronic pain, and mood disturbances.

Real-life Example:

- Peter, a 47-year-old IT consultant, had been suffering from digestive issues for years, including bloating, irregular bowel movements, and frequent fatigue. He also experienced significant mood swings and anxiety. After consulting a nutritionist, Peter discovered that his diet was contributing to an imbalance in his gut microbiome. By making dietary changes—such as eliminating processed foods and incorporating more fiber-rich, fermented foods—Peter noticed significant improvements in both his digestion and mood. His anxiety levels decreased, and he felt more mentally clear and focused.

3. The Hidden Cost of Ignoring Chronic Stress

Ignoring chronic stress can have devastating effects on both mental and physical health, particularly as men age. The emotional burden of unresolved stress not only affects the body's ability to function optimally but also impacts overall life satisfaction and quality of life.

Chronic Stress and Long-Term Health Risks

- Cardiovascular Issues: Chronic stress leads to increased heart rate and high blood pressure, which can contribute to long-term cardiovascular diseases, including heart attacks, stroke, and hypertension. The continuous cycle of stress and cortisol production wears down the body's ability to repair itself, leading to increased risk of heart-related issues.

- Immunosuppression: Stress weakens the immune system by impairing the production of white blood cells, which are responsible for fighting off infections. A chronically stressed individual is more susceptible to illness, infections, and diseases, as their body's natural defenses are weakened.

- Psychological Consequences: Ignoring chronic stress can lead to burnout, anxiety, and depression. Men who are emotionally overwhelmed but fail to address the underlying stress may experience diminished motivation, feelings of hopelessness, and difficulty managing their emotions.

Real-life Example:

- Frank, a 50-year-old business owner, ignored the signs of chronic stress for years. His work schedule was relentless, and he often felt overwhelmed but didn't seek help. Over time, his stress led to heart palpitations, chronic fatigue, and a noticeable drop in his mental health. It wasn't until he experienced a mild heart attack that he was forced to confront the toll his stress had taken. After this wake-up call, Frank worked with a therapist, started exercising regularly, and implemented better time management practices at work. His overall health and emotional resilience greatly improved as a result.

Conclusion

The mind and body are deeply interconnected, and the physical symptoms we experience are often the body's way of signaling emotional or psychological distress. Listening to these signals and addressing the root causes of chronic stress, gut health issues, and inflammation is crucial for maintaining both mental clarity and physical vitality. By paying attention to the subtle cues our bodies provide, men can take proactive steps toward improving their emotional and physical well-being.

Ignoring these symptoms can lead to long-term consequences for mental and physical health. By embracing a holistic approach that incorporates stress management, diet, exercise, and emotional awareness, men can create a stronger, healthier, and more resilient version of themselves—one that thrives both emotionally and physically in the second half of life.

CHAPTER 13

ADDICTION, NUMBING, AND THE DISTRACTIONS OF ESCAPE

Introduction: The Illusion of Escape

I n a world that demands constant output and offers constant distraction, it's not surprising that many men in midlife turn to escape mechanisms to cope with the mounting pressures of life. Whether it's a drink at the end of the day, endless scrolling through social media, or other forms of avoidance, these behaviors provide a temporary reprieve from the weight of responsibility, emotional discomfort, or stress. However, over time, these seemingly harmless activities can spiral into addiction, leading to numbing of emotions and disconnecting from real-life engagement.

This chapter will explore how seemingly benign coping mechanisms, such as drinking or excessive use of technology, can become dangerous forms of escapism. We'll dive into how these behaviors often act as short-term solutions for long-term emotional and psychological challenges and how they can undermine emotional growth, health, and relationships.

While these escape mechanisms might initially seem like they offer a reprieve, they only serve to postpone the deeper work needed to confront the underlying issues. The path to recovery doesn't necessarily require total abstinence or complete denial of pleasures but involves embracing mindful moderation and sober curiosity. We'll look at how men in midlife can replace escape with more engaging and healthy coping strategies that lead to real growth, well-being, and emotional connection.

1. When "Just a Drink" or Endless Scrolling Becomes a Coping Mechanism

The Subtle Slide into Escapism

In many social settings, alcohol or social media can start as harmless, enjoyable activities. A beer with friends, a glass of wine to wind down after a long day, or checking in with the world on social media for a few minutes can seem normal. But, as with many habits, these activities can easily slip into coping mechanisms.

For many men, these behaviors serve as temporary distractions from stress, boredom, or emotional pain. The issue arises when these distractions become habitual, and the emotional numbing becomes a way of life. Over time, the brain starts to rely on these activities to soothe itself, pushing away uncomfortable emotions or situations. Rather than confronting the emotional or psychological root causes of discomfort, men find themselves in a constant loop of escape—whether through substances or screen time.

The Role of Alcohol in Numbing and Avoidance

Alcohol is a common coping mechanism. A drink after work, a few beers during a social event, or a glass of wine while watching TV are ways that many men temporarily unwind or cope with stress. However, alcohol, even in moderate amounts, can begin to function as an escape mechanism for those dealing with anxiety, burnout, or personal challenges.

- Social Drinking: The socially accepted nature of drinking can make it difficult to recognize when it has transitioned from a social activity to a coping strategy. Men often face significant societal pressures to maintain an image of strength, control, and composure. When emotions are suppressed or ignored, alcohol can become the go-to solution for stress relief.

- The Escalation of Drinking Habits: While one or two drinks a night might seem harmless, drinking more frequently or in larger quantities over time can become problematic. As men age, the physical toll of alcohol can manifest in poorer sleep, digestive issues, and mood swings, all of which compound the reasons for continued drinking, creating a cycle of emotional numbing and poor self-care.

Real-life Example:

- Mike, a 46-year-old accountant, had been drinking a couple of beers every evening to "relax" after a stressful day at work. Over time, he began noticing that he was drinking more frequently, and the evenings began to revolve around it. What started as a few beers on Friday night turned into a daily ritual. His sleep suffered, and his energy levels were low. He realized he was using alcohol to numb the stress and anxiety that he hadn't dealt with. Once he acknowledged the issue, Mike started to explore ways of managing stress without relying on alcohol.

The Trap of Endless Scrolling

Social media has become another ubiquitous escape for men in midlife. What begins as harmless entertainment or a way to keep up with friends can morph into hours of mindless scrolling that distracts from real-life problems or emotions. Social media provides an instant dopamine hit—likes, comments, shares—but over time, it becomes less about connection and more about avoidance.

- The Emotional Numbing of Social Media: Social media is designed to grab attention and keep users engaged. However, spending excessive time scrolling can cause a person to disconnect from their own emotions, essentially "numbing" themselves to the reality of their life. Instead of facing personal difficulties, men may use social media to temporarily escape and live vicariously through other people's stories.

- The Comparison Trap: The downside of social media is the tendency to compare one's life to others, often leading to feelings of inadequacy, loneliness, or self-doubt. This can trigger more anxiety and stress, driving men to escape further into social media, creating a cycle of emotional avoidance.

Real-life Example:

- David, a 50-year-old tech executive, found himself spending hours each day scrolling through social media, especially at night when he was feeling stressed or bored. This habit began to take away from his real-life connections, as he felt disconnected from those around him. He realized that social media had become a way to avoid dealing with the emotional strain from his job and family responsibilities. Once David recognized the issue, he made a conscious effort to limit screen time and reconnect with friends and family through more meaningful interactions.

2. Replacing Escape with Engagement

The Importance of Emotional Engagement

Instead of relying on external distractions, men can benefit from engaging with their emotions directly. Emotional engagement means confronting feelings of stress, anger, frustration, and sadness head-on, rather than pushing them aside or numbing them with unhealthy coping mechanisms. This engagement often involves self-reflection, journaling, mindfulness, and communication.

The first step in replacing escape with engagement is to recognize that feelings, no matter how uncomfortable, are a natural part of life. Rather than avoiding or suppressing these emotions, engage with them. Acknowledge how you feel, accept it, and then explore healthy ways to process it.

Building Emotional Awareness and Mindfulness

- Mindfulness Practices: Mindfulness meditation, which focuses on being present and aware of your thoughts, feelings, and body, is a powerful tool for emotional engagement. It allows you to sit with uncomfortable emotions and process them without the need to escape or suppress them.

- Journaling: Writing down your thoughts and feelings is a therapeutic way to express emotions. By making a habit of journaling, men can begin to identify patterns in their emotional responses and start to understand the triggers that lead them to seek escape behaviors.

- Talking it Out: Open, honest communication with close friends, family, or a therapist can help men engage with their emotions in a constructive way. Verbalizing thoughts and feelings can reduce their intensity and make them feel more manageable.

Engagement Through Healthy Habits

- Physical Activity: Instead of turning to alcohol or social media, replace escape with activities that engage both the body and mind. Exercise, for instance, serves as a powerful way to manage stress, improve mood, and release pent-up tension. A regular workout routine or outdoor activities like hiking or cycling can provide a healthier outlet for stress.

- Creative Expression: Hobbies like art, music, or writing can offer an avenue for emotional expression. These activities allow men to channel their emotions into creative outlets, which can be both therapeutic and fulfilling.

- Engagement with Nature: Spending time in nature, whether through hiking, gardening, or simply walking in a park, can help men connect with their emotions in a grounding and healing way. Nature provides a sense of perspective and can act as a buffer against the overwhelming pressures of daily life.

3. The Path to Sober Curiosity or Mindful Moderation

Exploring Sober Curiosity

"Sober curiosity" is a relatively new term, but it's gaining traction as more people are beginning to question their relationship with alcohol. Instead of jumping into complete sobriety, sober curiosity allows men to explore their drinking habits without judgment or pressure. It's about developing a mindful awareness of alcohol consumption and its effects on both the body and mind.

- Mindful Drinking: Instead of mindlessly drinking to escape, mindful drinking is about being present and intentional with your choices. This means evaluating why you're drinking, how much you're drinking, and how it makes you feel. Are you drinking to numb an emotion, or are you drinking to enjoy a moment?

- Alternatives to Alcohol: Exploring non-alcoholic beverages or activities that don't revolve around drinking can help create new rituals of engagement. For example, instead of meeting friends at the bar, suggest a hike, coffee shop visit, or dinner without alcohol. This allows men to explore new ways of socializing without relying on alcohol.

The Benefits of Moderation

For those who aren't ready to commit to complete sobriety, mindful moderation is a healthy alternative. This approach involves setting clear boundaries around drinking and monitoring consumption to ensure it doesn't become a coping mechanism.

- Setting Boundaries: Establishing personal limits—such as only drinking on weekends or limiting the number of drinks per sitting—can help prevent alcohol from taking control. Being aware of one's own patterns and triggers can help maintain balance.

- Reflecting on the Why: Ask yourself why you drink and what you hope to gain from it. If you can find healthier ways to fulfill that need (e.g., stress relief, social connection), it may help reduce the reliance on alcohol.

Real-life Example:

- Chris, a 49-year-old sales manager, had spent many years relying on alcohol to manage stress after work. After exploring the idea of sober curiosity, he decided to cut back on alcohol and spent a month experimenting with not drinking on weekdays. He found that his energy levels were higher, his mood improved, and he slept better. This experiment led to a more mindful approach to drinking, where he now reserves alcohol for special occasions and avoids using it as a crutch for emotional escape.

Conclusion

Midlife is a time of reflection and recalibration, and it's a critical moment for men to evaluate their habits and behaviors, particularly when it comes to coping mechanisms. The temptation to escape through alcohol, social media, or other numbing behaviors is strong, but these temporary solutions can lead to deeper emotional and physical consequences over time. Instead, by replacing escape with engagement, mindful moderation, and sober curiosity, men can build healthier, more authentic coping strategies.

The goal is not to demonize drinking or social media, but to encourage a shift toward mindful self-awareness and the intention to engage with life in a more meaningful way. By reconnecting with the body and mind, exploring healthier habits, and being curious about the effects of alcohol, men can create a path toward greater emotional clarity, resilience, and well-being.

CHAPTER 14

THERAPY ISN'T WEAK – IT'S TACTICAL SELF-MASTERY

Introduction: Rewriting the Narrative of Mental Health

For many men, especially those over 40, mental health often remains a taboo subject—something to be avoided or ignored. Society has long conditioned men to perceive vulnerability as a sign of weakness and to suppress their emotions in the name of strength. This has resulted in an aversion to therapy, counseling, or any form of emotional support that might be perceived as "needy" or "weak." Yet, the reality is that therapy is not a sign of weakness; it is a strategic tool for personal growth and emotional self-mastery.

In midlife, many men face a growing realization that traditional models of strength—tied to stoicism, emotional suppression, and self-reliance—are no longer serving them. The challenges of aging, career changes, family dynamics, and health concerns are intense and require a new kind of strength: the strength to confront, process, and manage emotions in a healthy way. Therapy is not a crutch but a tactical tool that can help men unlock their true potential, achieve mental clarity, and create a life aligned with their core values.

This chapter will focus on dismantling the stigma surrounding therapy, presenting it as a powerful tool for men over 40 to achieve emotional well-being and resilience. It will provide guidance on how to find the right therapeutic fit—whether through therapists, coaches, or support groups—and outline a mental fitness plan that includes setting goals, tracking progress, and maintaining mental health.

1. Getting Past the Stigma: Therapy as a Tool, Not a Crutch

The Stigma of Therapy for Men

For much of history, men have been taught to tough it out, keep a stiff upper lip, and deal with challenges on their own. This has led to a deep societal stigma about seeking professional help for emotional or mental health issues. Therapy has often been viewed as something only weak people need or a last resort for those who cannot "handle" their problems.

In reality, therapy is a tool—a strategy for emotional self-mastery. The greatest leaders, athletes, and high performers often work with coaches or therapists to refine their skills, sharpen their minds, and overcome obstacles. The difference between those who succeed and those who struggle is often the ability to seek guidance, reflect on one's thoughts and emotions, and develop strategies for growth. Therapy is a proactive approach to taking control of one's mental and emotional well-being, not a passive crutch to lean on when things go wrong.

Therapy as Tactical Self-Mastery

Mental health is just as important as physical health, and investing in emotional well-being is no different from working on your fitness. Just as men work on physical strength through weightlifting or cardiovascular exercise, they can work on mental resilience through therapy. Therapy provides men with the tools to identify mental barriers, process emotions, and manage stress in a healthy way.

Therapy helps individuals build emotional intelligence, a skill that enables them to understand, manage, and express emotions effectively. By learning emotional regulation, men can face challenges with greater clarity, focus, and resilience. Therapy can also aid in overcoming negative thought patterns, such as anxiety, depression, or self-doubt, allowing men to create healthier relationships with themselves and others.

Therapy Is an Investment in Yourself

Therapy isn't just for when things go wrong—it is an ongoing practice of self-awareness and self-improvement. It's about becoming the best version of yourself. By prioritizing therapy as a regular part of life, men can make preventative mental health a priority rather than waiting for problems to escalate into crises. Therapy can serve as a preventive tool to maintain mental well-being, much like regular exercise maintains physical health.

Real-life Example:

- John, a 47-year-old executive, struggled with the pressures of a high-stress job, family life, and health concerns. Initially, he resisted therapy because he believed that it wasn't something "strong" men needed. However, after experiencing burnout and emotional exhaustion, he decided to give therapy a try. Over time, he began to see significant improvements in his emotional regulation, stress management, and overall mental clarity. By addressing his emotional challenges proactively, John was able to navigate midlife with a stronger sense of purpose and resilience.

2. How to Find the Right Fit: Coaches, Therapists, and Groups

Understanding the Different Types of Support

When it comes to seeking emotional support, there is no one-size-fits-all approach. Men can choose from a variety of mental health professionals based on their needs, goals, and personal preferences. The key is finding someone who understands the unique challenges of midlife and can offer practical, actionable strategies for emotional growth.

- Therapists and Counselors: Licensed therapists and counselors, such as clinical psychologists, social workers, or marriage therapists, provide therapeutic approaches like cognitive-behavioral therapy (CBT), psychodynamic therapy, or emotion-focused therapy (EFT). They are trained to help men address a wide range of emotional and psychological issues, from stress and anxiety to relationship problems and grief. Therapists offer a safe, confidential space to process emotions and work through difficult experiences.

- Coaches: Coaches, particularly life coaches or executive coaches, work with men who are focused on personal development and achieving specific goals. While therapy is more focused on healing and emotional processing, coaching often centers on goal-setting, self-improvement, and performance. A coach can provide practical advice and guidance on how to manage emotions, improve relationships, and achieve personal and professional growth. Coaches may not provide the same depth of therapeutic support as licensed therapists, but they can be valuable for men looking to make focused changes in their lives.

- Support Groups: Sometimes the best support comes from other people who are going through similar experiences. Support groups provide a sense of community and shared understanding, making them a great option for men seeking connection and mutual support. Groups can be in-person or online and are often centered around specific issues, such as anger management, grief, or addiction recovery. Many men find comfort in knowing they are not alone in their struggles and can draw strength from the collective wisdom of others.

How to Choose the Right Professional

When searching for the right coach, therapist, or support group, it's important to consider a few key factors:

1. Compatibility: The relationship between you and your therapist or coach is the foundation of effective therapy. It's essential to find someone with whom you feel comfortable, respected, and understood. Many therapists offer initial consultations or discovery sessions, allowing you to gauge whether their approach aligns with your needs.

2. Specialization: Consider what kind of support you need. Are you seeking help with stress management, anger issues, or relationship dynamics? Some therapists specialize in certain areas, while coaches may focus on personal growth or career development.

3. Accessibility and Logistics: Accessibility is important. Look for professionals who are available when you need them and who offer flexible scheduling. Online therapy or coaching may be an option for men who have busy schedules or prefer remote services.

Real-life Example:

- Mike, a 42-year-old IT specialist, had been struggling with work-life balance and family stress. After a year of avoiding therapy because of the stigma around it, he decided to try online therapy. He found a therapist who specialized in stress management and workplace anxiety, which allowed Mike to work through his issues at his own pace. The ability to have virtual sessions during his lunch break helped Mike maintain consistency in therapy, and over time, he noticed a significant improvement in his stress levels.

3. Mental Fitness Plan: Goals, Progress, and Maintenance

Just as physical fitness requires commitment, effort, and maintenance, so too does mental fitness. Establishing a mental fitness plan is essential for achieving sustained emotional well-being and resilience, especially as men navigate the complexities of midlife.

Setting Mental Fitness Goals

- Clarity: To begin building mental fitness, it's important to first gain clarity about what you want to achieve. This may involve identifying areas of life where you're struggling—stress, anxiety, communication in relationships, or self-esteem. Set clear goals for what you want to improve, and approach these goals with intention and purpose.

- Realistic Expectations: It's crucial to set realistic and achievable goals. Mental health progress is not linear, and there will be setbacks along the way. Start with small, manageable steps—such as committing to one therapy session a week or practicing mindfulness for 10 minutes a day—and gradually build your mental fitness from there.

Tracking Progress and Evaluating Success

- Journaling: Keeping a journal is a powerful way to track emotional progress. Journaling can help you identify patterns in your emotions, thoughts, and behaviors, making it easier to pinpoint areas of growth. Reflect on your experiences after each therapy session or coaching conversation, and note any breakthroughs or challenges.

- Regular Check-ins: Schedule regular check-ins with yourself or with your therapist/coach to assess progress. These can be weekly or monthly and should focus on celebrating your wins and reassessing your goals. Remember, therapy and self-improvement are ongoing processes, and it's important to stay committed to the journey.

Maintenance: Making Therapy Part of Your Life

Once you've made progress in therapy, maintaining your emotional fitness becomes just as important as reaching your initial goals. Therapy doesn't stop when the main issue is resolved—it's an ongoing process of growth, self-awareness, and maintenance.

- Continuing Therapy: For some, continuing therapy on a less frequent basis (e.g., once a month) helps maintain emotional well-being and resilience. Check-ins with a coach or therapist can ensure that you're staying aligned with your goals and staying emotionally fit.

- Ongoing Growth: Developing emotional fitness requires a commitment to continuous self-reflection, learning, and growth. Make mental wellness a priority, just as you would prioritize physical fitness.

Real-life Example:

- Brad, a 49-year-old business owner, worked with a therapist to address his work-related stress and relationship difficulties. After several months of therapy, Brad felt much more in control of his emotions and was better able to communicate with his family. He maintained his progress by scheduling monthly therapy sessions for maintenance and by regularly practicing stress-reduction techniques, such as mindfulness and journaling.

Conclusion

Therapy is not a sign of weakness; it is a strategic tool for emotional self-mastery and personal growth. Men over 40 can benefit greatly from seeking out therapy, coaching, or support groups to address emotional challenges and maintain mental fitness. By redefining therapy as a tool for empowerment and proactive health, men can experience better emotional regulation, stronger relationships, and a greater sense of well-being. Therapy, along with a commitment to mental fitness, provides the foundation for living a more authentic, fulfilled life—one in which emotional strength is celebrated and nurtured just as much as physical strength.

CHAPTER 15

LEGACY, LEADERSHIP & LIVING WELL

Introduction

As high achievers, we often place immense importance on the professional legacy we leave behind—our achievements, titles, and accolades that are measured by external accomplishments. However, as we navigate recovery, growth, and the quest for a balanced, fulfilling life, we are invited to reconsider the type of legacy we wish to leave—not just in terms of career success, but in terms of the personal impact we have on others. The true measure of success is not found in our professional titles or the wealth we amass; rather, it lies in the emotional strength and stillness we cultivate and share with the world around us. In the end, the legacy we leave is shaped not only by the work we do but also by the kind of person we become in the process.

This chapter is about exploring what it means to leave a legacy that encompasses emotional strength, resilience, and wisdom, qualities that will resonate with and inspire future generations. It is about leadership that begins with leading ourselves—becoming role models who embody the values we wish to pass on. We will explore the type of man (or woman) you are becoming, how you can be a role model for the next generation, and how to leave a legacy that is grounded in emotional strength and stillness.

What Kind of Man Are You Becoming Now?

The question of what kind of person we are becoming is one that calls us to examine our inner growth, our personal values, and the way we show up in the world. For high achievers, the relentless pursuit of success can sometimes overshadow the more important question of character development. But as we recover from past struggles, face our vulnerabilities, and work to rebuild a healthier, more balanced life, we are forced to reckon with who we are becoming—not just in our careers, but in our personal lives and relationships.

Becoming the person you want to be requires intentionality and reflection. It requires identifying the traits and values that you want to cultivate—whether it's compassion, resilience, integrity, or humility—and making them the cornerstone of your life. Recovery, in this context, becomes more than just the absence of addiction or unhealthy behaviors; it becomes the active process of becoming someone who can handle life's challenges with grace, strength, and wisdom. It's about learning to live with authenticity and purpose rather than chasing external validation.

For example, Mark, a high-level executive who had struggled with alcohol addiction, came to a pivotal moment in his recovery. He realized that his professional success had come at the cost of his relationships and emotional well-being. Mark asked himself: What kind of man do I want to be now? The answer wasn't about more promotions, higher salaries, or more recognition. It was about becoming a man who was emotionally present, who had the courage to be vulnerable, and who prioritized his mental and physical health above all else.

As Mark committed to his recovery, he worked on becoming the person who could truly show up for his family, his colleagues, and his community. He embraced the journey of personal growth, dedicating himself to being a man who could balance ambition with emotional intelligence and clarity. In doing so, he wasn't just rebuilding his professional life—he was reshaping his character, his relationships, and his legacy.

In recovery, we have the opportunity to examine who we are at our core and decide what qualities we want to embody moving forward. The question, "What kind of man are you becoming?" is an invitation to reflect on your values, your actions, and your growth. It's about identifying the traits you want to cultivate and living with intention to become the person you aspire to be.

Being a Role Model for the Next Generation

The role of a leader extends far beyond the workplace—it extends into our homes, communities, and social circles. As high achievers, we often find ourselves in positions where our actions, attitudes, and behaviors influence others. Whether you're a parent, mentor, colleague, or friend, you have the opportunity to shape the lives of those around you, particularly the next generation.

Becoming a role model means showing others not just what success looks like, but what it looks like to navigate life with emotional strength, resilience, and clarity. For many high achievers, the desire to be a role model goes hand-in-hand with the desire to leave behind a positive impact on others. The most powerful way to lead the next generation is by demonstrating through your actions how to live well—not just professionally, but personally. By embodying emotional health, vulnerability, and self-awareness, you show others that it is possible to succeed without sacrificing integrity or well-being.

Take the example of Tom, a father and senior leader in a corporation, who had spent years chasing success at the cost of his personal life. When Tom entered recovery from burnout and alcohol addiction, he realized that he wanted to model a different kind of success for his children—one that prioritized emotional health, strong relationships, and personal fulfillment. Tom began to show his children that success wasn't just about titles or achievements, but about living with purpose, being kind, and maintaining balance. He began to spend more time with his family, focusing on being emotionally available and present. He became open with his children about the importance of mental health and recovery, creating an environment where they felt comfortable talking about their feelings and challenges.

Being a role model means living in a way that aligns with your values and demonstrating those values through your actions. It's about showing others how to lead with integrity, how to overcome adversity, and how to maintain emotional balance in the face of life's inevitable challenges. By becoming a role model, you not only enrich the lives of those around you but also contribute to building a healthier, more compassionate world for future generations.

Leaving a Legacy of Emotional Strength and Stillness

Legacy is often thought of in terms of material wealth, achievements, or societal impact. But for those in recovery, the most important legacy you can leave is one of emotional strength and stillness—qualities that are invaluable in a world that often prioritizes external success over internal well-being. Emotional strength is the ability to face life's challenges with resilience, grace, and clarity. Stillness, in this context, is not about inactivity but about the ability to maintain inner peace, even in the face of external chaos.

For high achievers, the pursuit of emotional strength and stillness requires a shift in priorities. It involves moving away from the constant need to "do more" and embracing the importance of being present, reflecting on your emotions, and nurturing your inner peace. It's about creating a space within yourself where you can weather life's storms without being swept away by them.

The legacy of emotional strength and stillness is built over time through consistent practice. It involves cultivating habits that support emotional well-being—such as mindfulness, meditation, therapy, exercise, and healthy relationships—while also learning to detach from external pressures and expectations. It means learning to say no to things that drain your energy and yes to things that nourish your soul. It's about embracing vulnerability, understanding your limits, and living authentically, without the need to prove anything to others.

Consider the example of Michael, a successful business owner who had spent much of his life chasing professional accolades. After entering recovery, Michael began to realize that his true legacy wouldn't be defined by the number of deals he closed or the revenue his company generated. Instead, he focused on building emotional strength within himself, creating an environment of peace and stillness in his personal life, and teaching his children the importance of emotional health. Michael's legacy became one of emotional resilience—a legacy built on being grounded, present, and connected to what truly mattered in life.

Leaving a legacy of emotional strength and stillness is not only a gift to those who come after you, but also a gift to yourself. It is a way to live authentically, without the constant drive for external validation, and to create a life that is deeply rooted in peace, clarity, and purpose.

Conclusion

The legacy you leave behind is not determined by the accolades you collect, the promotions you receive, or the wealth you accumulate—it is shaped by the person you become, the emotional strength you cultivate, and the peace you embody. For high achievers in recovery, the process of becoming the person you aspire to be is not only about personal healing but about setting an example for others, particularly the next generation.

Being a role model in recovery means showing others that it is possible to succeed while maintaining emotional well-being, leading with integrity, and prioritizing self-care. It means demonstrating that strength isn't about perfection, but about resilience, vulnerability, and growth. By living with emotional strength and stillness, you can create a legacy that goes beyond professional success and leaves a profound, lasting impact on the people and communities you touch.

Ultimately, living well—living with clarity, purpose, and emotional balance—is the most important legacy you can leave. It is the gift that keeps on giving, inspiring others to embrace the journey of personal growth and recovery and to build their own legacies grounded in emotional health, authenticity, and fulfillment.

STRONG, STILL, AND JUST GETTING STARTED

T he journey of personal growth, especially for men over 40, is often marked by moments of reflection, realization, and renewal. Over the course of this book, we've explored the importance of embracing emotional health, cultivating mental resilience, and forging deeper connections with ourselves and others. From breaking the stigma surrounding therapy to redefining strength and vulnerability, these chapters have laid the groundwork for a more authentic, purposeful, and emotionally resilient life in midlife and beyond.

As we have seen throughout these chapters, mental fitness is just as important as physical fitness. Taking care of one's emotional well-being is a proactive and strategic decision—one that doesn't simply benefit mental health but impacts physical health, relationships, and overall life satisfaction. Therapy, mindfulness, self-reflection, and emotional self-regulation are not signs of weakness; they are powerful tools for creating a life that is balanced, meaningful, and aligned with our values.

Midlife: A Time for Recalibration

The period between 40 and 50 is a pivotal time for men. It is often a period of recalibration, where the past meets the present, and decisions are made about how to approach the future. Many men begin to feel the pressures of aging, career transitions, family responsibilities, and personal challenges. This chapter of life can bring about burnout, existential questioning, and the inevitable confrontation with one's own mortality. However, it is also an opportunity to take stock, confront deep-rooted emotions, and lay the foundation for a life that is more aligned with personal desires and values.

Through self-awareness, vulnerability, and the understanding that true strength comes from facing life's challenges with emotional depth, men can navigate midlife in a way that leads to profound growth. It's a time to ask, "What kind of man am I becoming now?" and recognize that the answer lies in how you engage with your emotions, relationships, and purpose.

The Power of Therapy and Emotional Engagement

Throughout the book, we've explored the crucial role that therapy plays in emotional self-mastery. Therapy is a tool, not a crutch. It allows men to break through emotional barriers, manage stress, and unlock their potential for growth. Mental fitness—just like physical fitness—requires consistent effort and intention. Therapy offers men a chance to reconnect with their emotions, process past traumas, and build resilience for future challenges. It's a proactive step toward becoming the kind of man who can lead with clarity, purpose, and empathy.

Whether through individual therapy, coaching, or support groups, seeking help and investing in emotional well-being is not just for times of crisis; it is a strategic decision for a long-term, healthy, fulfilling life. Therapy provides men with the emotional tools they need to manage the complexities of midlife and beyond, ultimately empowering them to live intentionally and authentically.

Leadership Through Emotional Strength and Vulnerability

Being a leader, whether in the workplace or at home, requires more than just the ability to manage tasks or people. Leadership begins with leading oneself—with emotional clarity, self-regulation, and the strength to confront challenges head-on. For men over 40, leadership is about embracing both strength and vulnerability—recognizing that true leadership is not about showing no emotion but about leading with emotional intelligence and empathy.

Men who embrace emotional strength in midlife become role models not only for their families but for their communities and the generations to come. By being authentic and vulnerable, they show others how to lead with both heart and clarity—how to balance toughness with tenderness, and how to confront life's challenges with resilience and purpose.

Building a Legacy of Emotional Health and Stillness

The legacy that men leave behind is not solely defined by career success, financial achievements, or material possessions—it's defined by the impact they have on others, the values they impart, and the emotional strength they model. A legacy of emotional health, self-awareness, and personal growth is one that transcends generations. It teaches the next generation the importance of self-care, emotional resilience, and living with integrity.

Midlife is the perfect time to reassess what kind of legacy you want to leave behind. The choices you make today—how you take care of your emotional health, how you engage with your loved ones, and how you lead your life with authenticity—will shape the legacy you create. The strength to lead with both presence and purpose will leave a lasting impact on those you care about, and it will create a foundation for the future that is grounded in emotional strength, vulnerability, and integrity.

The Second Act: Just Getting Started

As you move into the second act of your life, it's essential to view this stage not as the beginning of the end, but as the beginning of a deeper, more meaningful journey. It's an opportunity to recalibrate, to build on the lessons learned, and to continue growing emotionally, physically, and spiritually. Midlife is not a time to slow down; it's a time to lean into the possibilities that come with emotional self-awareness, strength, and purpose.

The second act is about more than just holding on to the past; it's about creating a life of fulfillment, meaning, and growth. The man you are becoming today—the one who values emotional fitness, embraces vulnerability, and lives with purpose—is the man who will thrive in the second half of life. Strength is not the absence of emotions; it's the presence of purposeful engagement with those emotions. Stillness is not about avoidance; it's about being grounded and connected to your own inner peace while navigating life's challenges.

The journey of becoming the best version of yourself continues, and as you step into the next phase, know that your second act starts here—with a commitment to emotional health, mindful living, and a legacy that will endure for years to come.

www.ingramcontent.com/pod-product-compliance
Lightning Source LLC
Chambersburg PA
CBHW070120030426
42335CB00016B/2219